confessions of a
veterinary nurse

Paws, Claws, and
PUPPy dog tails

Tracey Ison

Illustrations by Elspeth Rose Design

The Hubble & Hattie imprint was launched in 2009 and is named in memory of two very special Westies owned by Veloce's proprietors. Since the first book, many more have been added to the list, all with the same underlying objective: to be of real benefit to the species they cover, at the same time promoting compassion, understanding and respect between all animals (including human ones!)

Hubble & Hattie is the home of a range of books that cover all-things animal, produced to the same high quality of content and presentation as our motoring books, and offering the same great value for money.

Hubble & Hat

More great Hubble & Hattie books!

Among the Wolves: Memoirs of a wolf handler (Shelbourne)
Animal Grief: How animals mourn (Alderton)
Babies, kids and dogs – creating a safe and harmonious relationship (Fallon & Davenport)
Because this is our home ... the story of a cat's progress (Bowes)
Bonds – Capturing the special relationship that dogs share with their people (Cukuraite & Pais)
Camper vans, ex-pats & Spanish Hounds: from road trip to rescue – the strays of Spain (Coates & Morris)
Canine aggression – how kindness and compassion saved Calgacus (McLennan)
Cat and Dog Health, The Complete Book of (Hansen)
Cat Speak: recognising & understanding behaviour (Rauth-Widmann)
Charlie – The dog who came in from the wild (Tenzin-Dolma)
Clever dog! Life lessons from the world's most successful animal (O'Meara)
Complete Dog Massage Manual, The – Gentle Dog Care (Robertson)
Confessions of a veterinary nurse: paws, claws and puppy dog tails (Ison)
Detector Dog – A Talking Dogs Scentwork Manual (Mackinnon)
Dieting with my dog: one busy life, two full figures ... and unconditional love (Frezon)
Dinner with Rover: delicious, nutritious meals for you and your dog to share (Paton-Ayre)
Dog Cookies: healthy, allergen-free treat recipes for your dog (Schöps)
Dog-friendly gardening: creating a safe haven for you and your dog (Bush)
Dog Games – stimulating play to entertain your dog and you (Blenski)
Dog Relax – relaxed dogs, relaxed owners (Pilguj)
Dog Speak: recognising & understanding behaviour (Blenski)
Dogs just wanna have Fun! Picture this: dogs at play (Murphy)
Dogs on Wheels: travelling with your canine companion (Mort)
Emergency First Aid for dogs: at home and away Revised Edition (Bucksch)
Exercising your puppy: a gentle & natural approach – Gentle Dog Care (Robertson & Pope)
For the love of Scout: promises to a small dog (Ison)
Fun and Games for Cats (Seidl)
Gods, ghosts, and black dogs – the fascinating folklore and mythology of dogs (Coren)
Helping minds meet – skills for a better life with your dog (Zulch & Mills)
Home alone – and happy! Essential life skills for preventing separation anxiety in dogs and puppies (Mallatratt)
Know Your Dog – The guide to a beautiful relationship (Birmelin)
Letting in the dog: opening hearts and minds to a deeper understanding (Blocker)
Life skills for puppies – laying the foundation for a loving, lasting relationship (Zuch & Mills)
Lily: One in a million! A miracle of survival (Hamilton)
Living with an Older Dog – Gentle Dog Care (Alderton & Hall)
Miaow! Cats really are nicer than people! (Moore)
Mike&Scrabble – A guide to training your new Human (Dicks & Scrabble)

Mike&Scrabble Too – Further tips on training your Human (Dicks & Scrabble)
My cat has arthritis – but lives life to the full! (Carrick)
My dog has arthritis – but lives life to the full! (Carrick)
My dog has cruciate ligament injury – but lives life to the full! (Häusler & Friedrich)
My dog has epilepsy – but lives life to the full! (Carrick)
My dog has hip dysplasia – but lives life to the full! (Häusler & Friedrich)
My dog is blind – but lives life to the full! (Horsky)
My dog is deaf – but lives life to the full! (Willms)
My Dog, my Friend: heart-warming tales of canine companionship from celebrities and other extraordinary people (Gordon)
Office dogs: The Manual (Rousseau)
One Minute Cat Manager: sixty seconds to feline Shangri-la (Young)
Ollie and Nina and ... daft doggy doings! (Sullivan)
No walks? No worries! Maintaining wellbeing in dogs on restricted exercise (Ryan & Zulch)
Partners – Everyday working dogs being heroes every day (Walton)
Puppy called Wolfie – a passion for free will teaching (Gregory)
Smellorama – nose games for dogs (Theby)
Supposedly enlightened person's guide to raising a dog (Young & Tenzin-Dolma)
Swim to recovery: canine hydrotherapy healing – Gentle Dog Care (Wong)
Tale of two horses – a passion for free will teaching (Gregory)
Tara – the terrier who sailed around the world (Forrester)
Truth about Wolves and Dogs, The: dispelling the myths of dog training (Shelbourne)
Unleashing the healing power of animals: True stories about therapy animals – and what they do for us (Preece-Kelly)
Waggy Tails & Wheelchairs (Epp)
Walking the dog: motorway walks for drivers & dogs revised edition (Rees)
When man meets dog – what a difference a dog makes (Blazina)
Wildlife photography – saving my life one frame at a time (Williams)
Winston ... the dog who changed my life (Klute)
Wonderful walks from dog-friendly campsites throughout the UK (Chelmicka)
Worzel Wooface: For the love of Worzel (Pickles)
Worzel Wooface: The quite very actual adventures of (Pickles)
Worzel Wooface: The quite very actual Terribibble Twos (Pickles)
Worzel Wooface: Three quite very actual cheers for (Pickles)
You and Your Border Terrier – The Essential Guide (Alderton)
You and Your Cockapoo – The Essential Guide (Alderton)
Your dog and you – understanding the canine psyche (Garratt)

Hubble & Hattie Kids!

Fierce Grey Mouse (Bourgonje)
Indigo Warrios: The Adventure Begins! (Moore)
Lucky, Lucky Leaf, The: A Horace & Nim story (Bourgonje & Hoskins)
Little house that didn't have a home, The (Sullivan & Burke)
Lily and the Little Lost Doggie, The Adventures of (Hamilton)
Wandering Wildebeest, The (Coleman & Slater)
Worzel goes for a walk! Will you come too? (Pickles & Bourgonje)
Worzel says hello! Will you be my friend? (Pickles & Bourgonje)

www.hubbleandhattie.com

First published in June 2019 by Veloce Publishing Limited, Veloce House, Parkway Farm Business Park, Middle Farm Way, Poundbury, Dorchester, Dorset, DT1 3AR, England. Tel 01305 260068/fax 01305 250479/e-mail info@hubbleandhattie.com/web www.hubbleandhattie.com. ISBN: 978-1-787112-95-7 UPC: 6-36847-01295-3. © Tracey Ison & Veloce Publishing Ltd 2019. All rights reserved.
Readers with ideas for books about animals, or animal-related topics, are invited to write to the editorial director of Veloce Publishing at the above address. British Library Cataloguing in Publication Data - A catalogue record for this book is available from the British Library. Typesetting, design and page make-up all by Veloce Publishing Ltd on Apple Mac. Printed and bound in India by Replika Press PTY

confessions of a
veterinary nurse

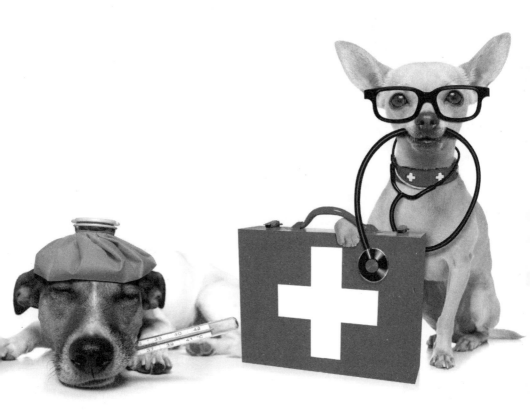

Paws, claws, and PUPPY dog tails

Tracey Ison

Hubble &Hattie

Dedicated to my wonderful husband, family and friends, both two and four-legged, for always believing.

Also, to Scout, my clumsy, flat-footed canine muse, for being my most honest critic.

And to the veterinary nurses, past, present and future: always be guided by your heart.

Contents

Forewords

Fascinating stories and a real insight into this profession, which has a public face and a coal face reality. Lots of humour and 'I can't believe it' moments.

All vet nurses, would be vet nurses, anyone who has worked back or front of house in a vet practice will love this, because THIS IS HOW IT IS!

Dr SDJ Marston BVetMed MF Hom MRCVS

Take a vicarious veterinary journey as you experience the trials, tribulations and 'tails' that helped forge an auspicious veterinary nursing career.

Tracey lets you into her head and heart to discover the passion and commitment that drove her to become a dedicated veterinary professional. Tracey delightfully weaves together the stories of early practice life, embracing the highs and lows of this unique vocation.

It is also a reminder to all animal carers and veterinary staff, when the days seem darkest, of that warm spark that was ignited in us in the first place, allowing us to do what we do, and turning a job into a way of life.

It is a privilege to have worked with Tracey, and to now be known as a friend.

Beautifully written. More to come, please.

David Edwards RVN

Introduction

Have I ever looked into the eyes of an animal who is sick or in pain and wondered if I could be the one to help, the one to make a difference?

Could I maintain a cool head in the face of a crisis, think fast, and act quickly?

Could I resist the urge to cry tears of joy at the birth of each new life?

Could I remain strong and hold back the tears, cradling a precious life in my hands as that life slipped away?

Were my shoulders strong enough to carry the heavy burden of emotional weight that came with devoting my life to caring for God's beautiful creatures?

These questions and more are asked by many veterinary nurses at some point during their careers, and what follows are the tales that always made me answer yes to every one.

Dreams can come true

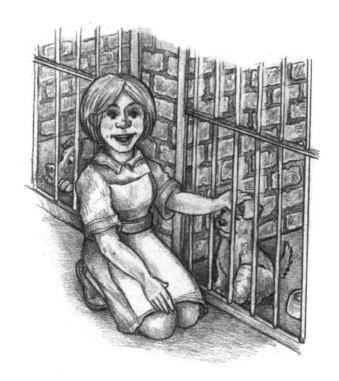

"**O**ne day," I mused, pausing momentarily to hitch my bag onto my shoulder, and turning to look at the imposing building I passed every day on my way to sixth form college.

The object of my attention was a veterinary practice. It was a stately, three-storey, Victorian building, with its ground floor fronted by a large set of bay windows. To one side was a large oak door set inside a recessed porch.

It was that door, and what was behind it, that I felt sure would be the way to my future, to all my dreams and aspirations.

You see, I loved animals - animals of all shapes and sizes; anything covered in fur, feather or scales would be guaranteed to set my heart fluttering.

As a child, I grew up alongside cats, dogs, rabbits, guinea pigs, and even a pair of gerbils at one point, whose escapology skills kept me entertained for hours. If I wasn't petting, stroking or cuddling an animal, I was writing about them, creating a personal mini-library of notebooks filled with the adventures of fictitious animals whose characters I brought to life inside the colourful labyrinth of my imagination.

I had dreamt of working with animals for as long as I could remember. I envisaged a career spent ministering to sick animals, helping to ease suffering and provide comfort, love, and, of course, an endless supply of cuddles; being able to hold a paw during a time of crisis seemed to be the only way forward for me.

Advancing through my teenage years in the mid-1980s, I began to consider the various career options that centred around animal care. I wondered about studying to be a vet, but I was daunted by the long list of qualifications required, and the many years of training involved. I considered myself to be reasonably academic, but that career path did seem to be a little too far out of my reach. With that notion well and truly put aside, I dug a little deeper and began to investigate the role of a veterinary nurse.

During the eighties, qualified veterinary nurses in the UK were known as Animal Nursing Auxiliaries or ANAs (prior to this they had the slightly longer title of Registered Animal Nursing Auxiliaries). To qualify as an ANA you had to secure a training position at a veterinary practice and complete a two-year training course, with an exam at the end of each year comprising three parts: written, oral, and practical. Most of the training was done on the job, and all trainees enrolled on the course were issued with a training book. This little green book contained a list of practical skills, in which the trainee would have to achieve a high level of competency before being signed off by a senior vet. The tasks in the book were numerous, and varied from simple sounding exercises (such as cleaning out a kennel) to more complex ones: for example, applying a bandage or administering an injection. At the end of the two-year training course, the training book had to be fully completed and signed off, demonstrating that the trainee had received adequate training and was competent enough to carry out a range of practical nursing tasks.

This all sounded perfect to me, but there was a snag – a pretty big snag.

Trainee veterinary nurse positions were scarce, and vacancies were rare. In our town, there were only two veterinary practices, and I guess I was one of countless animal lovers all waiting for a golden opportunity to secure their dream job. If ever there was even the slightest whiff of a vacancy, scores and scores of people would apply.

Still, it pays never to give up on a dream, and sometimes just being in the right place at the right time can change your life forever; it just so happened that I found the 'right place.'

For me, it was the sixth form common room, one morning back in November 1986. Every morning, before classes started, students were encouraged to gather in the central common room to listen to the head form tutor, Mr Stoker, read out school notices, and remind students of various school activities, etc. It was all quite informal, and attendance was voluntary. On that morning, I was toying with the idea of giving it a miss. I'd got one of the best seats in the classroom – comfortably ensconced, warming my back against a radiator – but I was persuaded by my friends to tag along, so I, somewhat begrudgingly, joined the throng.

I half listened as Mr Stoker rattled through some notices, but my ears pricked up when I heard the words 'local vets.' I could scarcely believe it. One of the local veterinary practices (the same one that I had been passing every day for years) had contacted Mr Stoker, looking to employ a student nurse. I thought I must have nodded off and been dreaming it all, until a sharp dig in the ribs from my best friend, Helen, convinced me otherwise.

confessions of a veterinary nurse

"That's it, Tracey," she whispered excitedly. "That's your job."

I could hardly wait until the announcements were over before scurrying over to Mr Stoker to ask for more information. It seemed that I was not the only one whose curiosity had been piqued, and I joined a long queue, waiting my turn to find out more. As soon as I reached him, I asked Mr Stoker what I needed to do next to apply for the position.

My mind was whirring with excitement; I could barely stop myself from snatching the letter from the veterinary practice, containing details of the job, straight from his hand.

"It's all written on here," he said. "Greenfield Veterinary Centre is looking to employ a full-time student nurse – in-house training will be provided, and the trainee will also be enrolled onto the nurse training scheme. Written applications will be considered, and interviews will follow for all suitable candidates. Bear with me and I'll write down the address for you."

"That's okay," I replied, with a wide smile. "I already know it."

I couldn't wait for my classes to end that day. I practically ran home, and, breathlessly, I spoke to my parents about the amazing job opportunity that had presented itself.

My parents have always been supportive, and they also knew this was something I was going to do no matter what, so with pen and paper at hand, I put together a letter of application and tucked it away in an envelope.

Mum offered to post it for me, but I was not going to leave something so precious in the hands of the postal system. No – there was only one way to ensure that this letter was delivered safely and that was to do it myself.

On my way to college the following morning, with my letter of application clutched firmly in my hand, I walked down the short driveway of Greenfield Vets, up to the big wooden door, and, with my free hand, I pushed it open.

I was instantly greeted by a warm rush of air and the heady smell of disinfectant. As I entered the waiting room, I let my eyes wander, taking in the spacious seating area, the rustic oak floor, the high ceilings with ornate cornices, and the tall filing cabinets, which I imagined held patient records.

"Hello there, how can I help?" A bright voice, belonging to a smiling, smartly-dressed lady, came from behind the reception desk.

"Hi," I replied. "I am dropping in my application for the position of trainee veterinary nurse."

"I will take it for you and pass it on to the practice principal," she said, plucking the letter from my outstretched hand and placing it on top of a large pile of envelopes, which I presumed were all from fellow applicants. "We'll start to process these soon, and there will be a shortlist of applicants who will be invited along for an interview. Good luck with your application."

All I could do now was wait …

A few days later, I received the news I'd been hoping for: I had been invited to attend an interview with the practice principal. I was excited, nervous, apprehensive, and on the morning of the interview I could hardly contain the butterflies in my stomach.

I was suitably attired, with the help of my mum, in a smart skirt and blouse, and felt very grown up as I sat waiting to be called to see the practice principal.

After about half an hour, I was summoned upstairs to meet Gerald Crossland, practice principal and owner of Greenfield Vets. This was it!

The first time I met Gerald (though I was never to call him by his first name to his face; he was always Mr Crossland), I was awestruck. In his mid-50s, Gerald had a genuine air of grandeur about him, clad in what I later came to acknowledge as a veterinary standard – a tweed jacket and brown corduroy trousers. (Don't ask me at what stage of veterinary training, students become obliged to wear tweed, but it seemed to be an industry-wide fashion statement). As he stood to greet me, I suddenly felt a little overwhelmed, and almost felt like dropping into a curtsey. I hastily quashed that notion, and reached out to shake the hand that had been offered to me.

"Ahh," he boomed, fixing me with a big smile and picking up my letter from the top of a stack, which was precariously balanced on one side of his desk. I did notice (it was difficult not to) that his desk was piled high with all sorts of letters, documents, and official looking forms. A little haphazard, it looked as if one of the piles of paperwork might topple over at any moment.

"Take a seat, Tracey." He gestured, peering at me over the top of the horn-rimmed glasses that framed his very dignified face, with its ruddy complexion, which I guessed reflected years of working outdoors.

I don't remember much about the interview; I spent most of it trying to control the wobble in my voice every time I answered a question. I tried to keep my mind focused by concentrating on the pieces of paper that Gerald was scribbling notes on as we talked. (I would find out many years later that Gerald, in fact, made no notes whatsoever during any interviews – he just doodled animals and trees).

Interview complete, Gerald gave me another firm handshake and advised me that someone would be in touch within a week. Stifling the urge to curtsey again, I took my leave and hurried away, hoping that I had managed to give the right impression.

I obviously did, because the following day I received a phone call: they were offering me the position of trainee veterinary nurse. I could hardly believe my luck!

An official letter arrived in the post shortly afterwards, confirming my start date: Monday 24 November 1986 at 9.00 am. My starting wage for a forty-hour week was to be the princely sum of a pound an hour (rising to the giddy heights of one pound fifty per hour overtime). I would be provided with a uniform, and enrolled onto the nurse training course as soon as I had completed the obligatory trial period.

The following couple of weeks were a whirlwind of activity, attending exit meetings from my college, filling in a mountain of paperwork, and saying goodbye to form tutors and school friends, most of whom would soon be moving away to university. Suddenly, it was becoming a reality: I was leaving the relative safety of further education and was going to become a worker, earning a wage and hopefully contributing something meaningful to the world. I couldn't wait.

My first day as a worker, I was up bright and early, and spent far too much time trying to decide what to wear and how I should do my hair. Mum eventually stepped in, choosing trousers and a jumper for me, and helping me scrape my often-unruly mane of red hair into a smart ponytail. After handing me a packed lunch, she waved me off, and I took the twenty-minute walk to my new place of employment.

Standing once more in front of the old oak door, I took a deep breath, drew myself up to my full five-foot height, and stepped over the threshold into a new life.

Sitting at the reception desk was the kind lady who had taken my application form a few weeks earlier.

"Hello again," she said brightly. "You must be Tracey? I'm Sarah, one of the receptionists here. Welcome aboard." She gave me such a warm smile that I felt some of my 'first day' nerves start to melt away.

"I will let Mr Crossland know that you are here. He should have remembered that today was your starting date." Sarah picked up the phone and began dialling. "I hope," she added under her breath.

Curious, I thought. Surely he would know that I was starting today. I shrugged my shoulders and took a seat.

After a short while, the reception telephone rang and Sarah picked it up. There was a short exchange of words, with Sarah saying, "yes, it was definitely today," before fixing me with a slightly embarrassed smile. "Mr Crossland is expecting you if you would like to pop upstairs, he will ... umm ... well, he will sort things out for you," she said breezily.

By now, I had the distinct impression that, while Sarah knew I was due to start today, Mr Crossland had forgotten all about it. How very odd, I thought. I took my leave, headed upstairs, and knocked on the office door.

"Come in, come in."

I opened the door and there was Mr Crossland, seated at his desk, still flanked on either side by untidy piles of paperwork.

"Ah, yes, it's Tina, isn't it?" he said, getting to his feet and striding towards me with an outstretched arm, ready for another firm handshake. He seemed oblivious to the fact he had inadvertently knocked over one of his precarious stacks of paper, merely walking over them as they fluttered to the ground.

"It's Tracey, actually," I replied. "Today is my first day."

"Of course, yes." He flashed me an apologetic grin. "I am terrible with names and dates and things, do forgive me. Well, first things first, let's get you a uniform." He strode out of the room and I trotted dutifully after him.

"Here we are," he said, opening a large wardrobe that stood just outside the office. After rummaging around for a few moments, he turned to me with a flourish and said, "I think this one should fit. If you would like to get changed, I'll go and find Jenny, our head nurse; she'll show you around."

I cringed inwardly at the garment Mr Crossland was holding out to me. I'd seen pictures of trainee nurses' uniforms in books - they were smart, green and white, pin-striped, knee-length dresses, with a classic white nurses' apron worn on top. This garment, however, looked like something befitting an Edwardian parlour maid. Fashioned from a dark green and white, tightly pin-striped, heavy-duty fabric, it had long sleeves that ballooned from the shoulders then narrowed to wide, buttoned cuffs at the wrist. Lengthwise, at a guess, I suspected it would reach mid-shin. It looked so old-fashioned that I wouldn't have batted an eyelid if it'd had a bustle at the back! After a little more rummaging, Gerald produced a slightly worn, elasticated white belt, and finally, thankfully, a crisp and almost-new nurse's apron. Bundling them into my arms, Gerald waved me off to the nearby bathroom to get changed, and wandered off, presumably to find Jenny.

Five minutes later, I had changed into my new uniform. There was no mirror in the bathroom, so I couldn't see how I looked, but I felt very conscious of the dress swishing around my lower legs as I made my way back down the stairs and out into reception.

Sarah was still at her post, but had been joined by another new face, who I took to be Jenny. Attired in the bottle green dress of a qualified nurse, sporting a similar white apron to my own, she came straight over to me.

"Hi." She smiled. "Sorry I wasn't here to greet you. Mr Crossland got his days a bit muddled and we were not expecting you until next week. I'm Jenny and I am the head nurse here. Come with me and I will show you around."

Jenny took me on a tour of the main building. Leading off from the reception area and waiting room were two consulting rooms. One was large and airy, with huge windows on two sides allowing the November morning sunlight to flood in. This, Jenny explained, was Mr Crossland's consulting room, and was not to be used by anyone else. It was the nurses' job, she added, to ensure that the consulting rooms were kept tidy and restocked daily. Jenny opened some of the cupboard doors to reveal a dizzying array of tablets, bottles of injectable liquids, syringes, needles, dressing materials, and other medical paraphernalia that I couldn't identify.

"Don't worry," she said. "We will give you full training on what's what in here, as well as how to clean and look after the equipment and instruments."

We moved into the second consulting room, which was a lot smaller, and used by one of Greenfield's current vets during consulting hours.

Down a long, narrow corridor we passed the large animal dispensary (a larder in years gone by), which was accessed by a sliding door. It was crammed from floor to ceiling with boxes, bottles, and tins of medications. Jenny assured me that I would soon become familiar with the range and variety of products that the practice stocked.

Next stop, after passing a third consulting room that led off the corridor, we came to the small animal pharmacy, a collection of tall cupboards that reached up to the ceiling, each one packed with different medications.

"It's the nurses' responsibility to order and maintain the stock in both the small and large animal pharmacies," explained Jenny. "It's easy enough to do once you get the hang of it: you just need to be pretty handy at using a set of stepladders to reach the top shelves."

We were now in the last room at the far end of the building. A tidy kitchen, with a sink and a very old gas oven and hob, on top of which stood a large, metal, cylindrical-shaped object that looked to me like a pressure cooker.

"This is our autoclave," Jenny said. "We sterilise all of our instruments, drapes and suchlike in it."

With the tour of the main building complete, we went outside, across the small driveway, and into the kennel and theatre building; Jenny described this building as the surgical unit.

Upon entering, I was once again mindful of the warmth and the strong smell of disinfectant.

confessions of a veterinary nurse

We passed a row of kennels, all fully occupied. Jenny paused to reach through the bars of one, to stroke the head of a little Labrador puppy whose front leg was encased in a large bandage.

"This is Harvey," she said quietly, as Harvey nuzzled at her hand. "Harvey had a tumble down a flight of stairs and broke his leg, poor boy. He's in today for a bandage change."

The kennel room led straight into the surgical preparation area. Jenny explained that all patients having surgical procedures were 'prepped' in this room, hence frequently referred to as prep rooms. Here, patients were checked and sedated prior to being anaesthetised. Then, the surgical sites were clipped, and the skin was cleaned by scrubbing with an appropriate skin disinfectant. Once done, the anaesthetised patient was then transferred to the sterile operating theatre ready for surgery.

The preparation area was a small space, filled in the most part by a centrally-located table, topped by a non-slip mat. An anaesthetic machine, with all sorts of pipes and tubing hanging off it, stood in one corner, and a desk was situated opposite, facing a large window that provided a clear view into the operating theatre.

The theatre itself was currently in use. One of the vets was bent over a patient, busily working away whilst the nurse stood to one side, stethoscope in her ears, a look of concentration on her face as she listened intently to the patient's breathing.

Both looked up momentarily and gave me a cheery wave.

"That is James, one of our vets." Jenny waved back. "And with him is Lucy, our qualified nurse. I will introduce you properly later. Follow me and I will show you our X-ray room."

The X-ray room was accessed via the prep area, and was essentially a converted garage. A row of wooden walk-in kennels flanked one side of the room, and on the other was the X-ray unit.

It was a huge piece of equipment – a large lead-lined table with an X-ray head above it. The on/off switch was an enormous lever bolted to the wall. I have to say, it reminded me of the type of machinery that would feature heavily in old black-and-white Frankenstein movies.

"It is quite dated," said Jenny, obviously picking up on my slightly worried expression. "A bit of a find, really. Mr Crossland heard that a local hospital was getting rid of it and offered to give it a new home. It's passed all its safety checks, but I admit it does look a bit scary. He loves a bargain, does Mr Crossland. Well, that's us, then," Jenny said, turning to face me. "What do you think?"

I was impressed by all that I had seen so far, if not a little overwhelmed, which is what I told her.

"You'll be just fine," she said, with an encouraging smile.

The rest of my day passed in a bit of a blur. Jenny and I sat in the office and went through my daily duties and responsibilities as a trainee, and my starting rota. James and Lucy both popped in to welcome me to the practice.

Before I knew it, it was 5 o'clock and time to go home. As I was preparing to leave, Jenny laid a hand on my shoulder and said, "it's okay, you can leave your uniform here. You don't have to walk home in it - it is a tad old-fashioned." I could tell she was trying to stifle a laugh, and I took her up on her offer; not once did I ever pluck up the courage to wear that particular uniform on my journey to and from work.

Visit Hubble and Hattie on the web:
www.hubbleandhattie.com • www.hubbleandhattie.blogspot.co.uk
Details of all books • Special offers • Newsletter • New book news

Monkey business

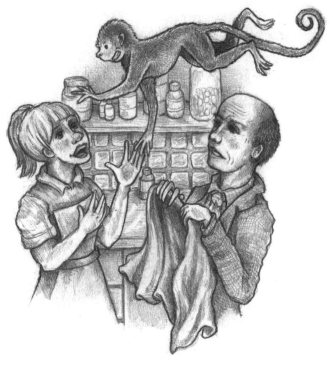

And so it began, life as a student veterinary nurse.

I quickly learnt that I was well and truly on the bottom rung of a very tall ladder, and that working my way up was going to be a hard slog.

During my first few weeks I cleaned. I cleaned a lot!

I started on syringe washing. Used syringes from around the practice were collected daily, in a large metal bowl that was left in the small animal pharmacy next to the sink. I had to fill the sink with a diluted solution of disinfectant (which was bright blue in colour), and, one by one, I took apart and washed every syringe, rinsing each one thoroughly before placing them in a clean bowl. Once I'd dried each one by hand with a paper towel, I had to put them back together again, pack them into special heatproof bags, then seal and sterilise them in the practice autoclave ready for re-use. Of course, these days, syringes are disposable, and discarded after a single use, but back then it was common practice to re-sterilise and reuse. You could always tell when I had just processed a large batch of syringes, as my hands and arms would be stained blue by the disinfectant, from the tips of my fingers right up to my elbows.

I also became chief surgical drape washer. Following surgical procedures, the green, heavy-duty, cloth drapes used to cover surgical sites were dropped into a bucket of cold water to help remove any blood that had soaked into them. Once full, I would collect the bucket and hand scrub the drapes until they were clean, before hanging them up to dry. Once dry and folded in a specific way, I packed and sealed them in heatproof bags, sterilising them in the autoclave. Used surgical kits also came my way, each one needing to be carefully hand cleaned, checked for damage, dried, and packaged correctly ready for sterilising.

I cleaned walls, floors, doors, and cupboards, inside and out. I soon became acquainted with a variety of different types of disinfectants and cleaners, their dilutions, and how they worked to keep the practice spotlessly clean and germ-free.

I didn't mind the cleaning jobs for the most part, as I took the opportunity to look at the things I was cleaning, trying to identify them and learn their uses. Luckily, there was always someone around to answer my many questions.

Another task I was given was 'bottling up' – decanting liquid medicines from large glass bottles into smaller ones for dispensing to patients. I had to ensure that they were all correctly labelled, and that the stock in the consulting rooms was regularly replenished. Cough mixtures, health tonics, shampoos, and kaolin-based 'bad tummy' concoctions were just some of those in regular use. The kaolin-based medicines were my least favourite: thick and gloopy in consistency, try as I might, I could rarely fill a bottle without the stuff getting everywhere.

Whilst working in the dispensary, I was often asked by the vets to count prescribed tablets into tablet bottles. Back then, there was a very limited range of medications available for domestic pets; antibiotics were mostly penicillin and tetracyclines, and most other medications fell into the broad categories of 'arthritis pills,' 'heart pills' or 'kidney pills.' Nevertheless, I enjoyed getting to know the names of each type of tablet and what their mode of action was.

The one thing I came to dread was dealing with the 'large animal' buckets. Whilst out on farm visits, the large animal vets, who attended farm animals and horses, accumulated a lot of waste – used syringes, instruments, soiled bandage materials, empty vaccine vials and injectable bottles, partly used boxes of medications, and other sundry items. Everything they used was deposited into large plastic buckets. The idea was that once a bucket was full, it was left in the pharmacy to be sorted and emptied. However, the vets tended to be a little remiss about bringing their full buckets in. Only when they ran out of space in their cars, would they remember to bring in their buckets – often several at once.

Some mornings I could tell there were a fresh collection of full buckets waiting for me because of the smell that emanated from the pharmacy. As I said, everything went in these buckets, including, on many occasions, generous dollops of manure (don't ask me how they managed to do this so frequently), various lumps of dried up animal tissue from minor surgical procedures, and other completely unidentifiable objects, usually all heavily encrusted with blood. The equipment that I expected to find would also be heavily soiled. Considering that the buckets had probably spent a good week or so in the boot of a car, it wasn't surprising that they developed a distinct aroma all of their own.

17

confessions of a veterinary nurse

Wearing gloves, I had to carefully empty each of the buckets in turn. Despite being equipped with special containers to dispose of used hypodermic needles, the vets would sometimes accidentally throw an uncapped syringe and needle into the bucket, making the job even worse, so taking care was especially important.

Still, there was always a great feeling of satisfaction when I looked at the gleaming row of empty, freshly-washed buckets all waiting to go back out with the vets.

From syringe washer and bucket scrubber, I quickly progressed to kennel cleaning, which took me where I really wanted to be - the surgical unit.

Kennel cleaning was an on-going process. A morning ward round was conducted by the early shift nurse, who would record her observations about any patients that had been in overnight. Observations included the patient's demeanour, if they had eaten or drunk, and if they had vomited or passed diarrhoea. The patient would be moved to a clean kennel while theirs was thoroughly cleaned and disinfected, before being transferred back. Once the kennels had all been cleaned, the vet on duty would join the nurse on the ward round to discuss treatment plans for each patient. Any patient who soiled their kennel during the day would require immediate cleaning, and each kennel was also cleaned after the patient was discharged.

Kennel cleaning gave me my first opportunity to interact with the patients. I couldn't wait to join Jenny or Lucy for their morning rounds; I shadowed them until they felt I was able to conduct the initial part of the ward round myself, before the vet attended.

Mostly, our patients were cats and dogs, but occasionally a rabbit, bird, or guinea pig could be found in the kennel blocks. As the small animal side of the practice was still growing, and overnight hospitalisation of patients was not very common, our inpatient numbers were small, usually no more than two or three on any given day.

As we removed each patient from their kennel - so it could be cleaned - we checked them over. Some patients soiled themselves overnight, and were, for the most part, grateful for a gentle bed bath to clean dirty paws and faces. Brushing our inpatients also helped to provide some one-to-one interaction with a friendly face. Dogs that were able to do so were walked around the back garden to give them a little fresh air, and cats were usually cuddled. Dirty food and water bowls, used cat litter trays and bedding were removed and replaced, and each kennel re-lined with newspaper (an excellent source of insulation, and very useful for soaking up the plethora of different waste products that were expelled by our patients) and a pad of comfortable, absorbent bedding.

I gained so much valuable experience from these early morning ward rounds. I learnt to correctly approach a nervous patient by avoiding eye contact, keeping my body posture quite low, and using a gentle tone of voice. I also learnt that gentle stroking around the chest and shoulders of a dog often had quite a calming effect, whereas rubbing a cat under their chin helped them relax and feel more at ease. I was taught how to recognise the tell-tale signs that indicate an animal might be in pain: a hunched posture, elevated breathing rate, or even signs of aggression in a normally friendly animal.

I was encouraged to handle the patients, and shown how to perform basic checks such as measuring heart, breathing, and pulse rates, and taking temperatures, not always the easiest thing to do when your patient is a wriggling ball of fluff who just wants to lick your face.

At the end of each shift, I would hurry home to study. There were limited reading resources available for student nurses, but there was one reference book that no student nurse could do without: *Jones's Animal Nursing*. Costing the equivalent of one week's wages, I was lucky enough to receive a copy from my parents at Christmas. Every night, I would sit in my bedroom and immerse myself in reading, scribbling notes as I studied each page intently.

The book contained everything I needed to know, from anatomy and physiology, to anaesthesia, bandaging techniques, first aid, and laboratory work – all the things I desperately wanted to put to practical use.

After my first two weeks at Greenfields, I was enrolled onto the veterinary nurse training course. Once a week, I had to attend college, one which was a considerable distance away. Because I couldn't drive, I caught the bus first thing in the morning, changing buses at a central depot halfway through the journey. The bus drivers soon got to know me, and allowed me to stay on the first bus to keep warm whilst waiting for the next one. The driver would bang on the side of the bus to let me know when my next bus arrived. I got into the habit of having a quick nap, and once or twice missed my connecting bus because the driver had forgotten to wake me up.

After a long day at college and a long journey back, I returned to work to finish the late shift, often not getting home until after eight o'clock.

Did this bother me? Not one bit. I was loving every minute.

Armed with my very own little green training book, I threw myself heart and soul into my work. Every day I learned something new, every day my knowledge expanded a little bit more.

I also got to know my colleagues, and forged many friendships that are still going strong today. There was, and still is, a great deal of camaraderie amongst veterinary professionals. The veterinary industry is a tough one, requiring a high level of commitment and teamwork. The vets and nurses I have worked alongside have always been dedicated and incredibly passionate about their chosen career path.

I soon discovered that Gerald Crossland, our practice principal, was a living legend in our town: a well-established sage when it came to the health and welfare of horses, and as such was always in great demand. Every morning he would sweep regally into reception, and those seated in the waiting room would stare at him in awe as he passed, making his way into his office.

Timekeeping wasn't Gerald's strong point, and his love of a strong cup of tea before he began his morning consultations always meant that he ran behind with his appointments. His waiting clients didn't seem to mind one bit; they all seemed to be under the impression that he must be otherwise engaged saving lives.

Gerald had a very lax attitude towards business. The untidy heaps of paperwork that adorned his desk never diminished in size, and consisted mostly of unpaid invoices. Both receptionists and nurses were adept at fielding calls from creditors, and I also became accustomed to seeing Gerald slipping quietly out of the back door whenever we received visits from suppliers or tradespeople demanding payment for goods and services.

If he was ever pinned down and had to face a creditor, Gerald always managed to charm himself an extension to his payment deadline.

Gerald chose not to interact on a personal level with his staff, and relied instead on writing messages in a diary for us to read. Sometimes he would stand right next to me, scribbling away, even when it would have been much easier to speak to me, but that was just his way.

Most of the time, all I got was a polite nod, and, if I was really honoured, maybe a good morning every now and then. It was usually one of the nurses who would take Gerald his morning and afternoon cup of tea, and try as I might, I never lost the desire to curtsey after placing a hot beverage on his desk. Instead, I took to slowly walking backwards away from him, fearing that turning my back on him would somehow be perceived as an act of disrespect.

Rarely did Gerald ask for help from one of the nursing team during his consultation sessions, but every now and then we were called to assist with a fractious or difficult patient.

One of the more difficult patients that Gerald asked me to help with was a poorly spider monkey he had been treating for a severe case of diarrhoea. A local client held a licence to keep exotic animals and was a frequent visitor with some of her more unusual pets.

The monkey, who was called Eric, was sitting forlornly on the bottom of his transport cage when I first entered the consulting room. Gerald was standing to one side of the cage, holding a large towel in his hands. Our plan was for Gerald to scoop up Eric in the towel, wrap him securely, and hand him to me, leaving Gerald free to examine him. As the little monkey looked very quiet and placid, obviously feeling very out of sorts, this seemed like a sensible way forward. Gerald opened the top of the transport cage, gently lowered the towel over Eric, and carefully lifted him out.

Eric, on the other hand, had a completely different idea in mind. With a sudden, ear-piercing shriek, Eric sprang to life and shot out of the towel before Gerald had the chance to contain him. Gerald, myself, and Eric's owner could only stand by and watch as Eric began hurtling around the consulting room. I ducked as Eric leapt over my head and landed on a window ledge before taking off again. He crashed into a set of shelves that were heavily laden with tablet bottles, medications, syringes, needles, and other veterinary supplies that, up until that moment, had all been very neatly arranged. The sound of it all hitting the floor was pretty much drowned out by Eric's high-pitched screeching.

What ensued was five minutes of sheer horror. As well as hurling himself wildly around the confines of the consulting room, Eric began to emit jets of foul-smelling liquid diarrhoea.

Gerald's usual unflappable, stiff-upper-lip countenance disintegrated into one of total dismay as the contents of Eric's bowels splashed and splattered all over his immaculate consulting room, coating the walls, tables, and cupboards. Eric's owner caught a very unpleasant offering that landed directly on top of her head and proceeded to trickle down her neck and shoulders like warm, brown lava.

Gerald tried valiantly to recapture Eric in the towel, shaking it at him in a style vaguely reminiscent of a matador, but Eric was having none of it, and simply sprang out of the way every time the towel was hurled in his direction.

I felt nothing but empathy for Gerald as a particularly savage expulsion of liquid faeces hit one of his most treasured possessions, a framed photograph of his wife receiving a handshake from the Queen at a well-known equine event. The beaming faces of Gerald's wife and Her Majesty quickly disappeared underneath a sticky coating of Eric's finest.

Those few minutes seemed to last for an eternity as all three of us ducked and dived to avoid Eric as he swooped around us, using the light fittings to swing himself onto the tops of cupboard and shelves, showering us with even more liquid faeces as he flew back and forth.

Eventually, Eric began to tire. He wasn't in tip-top health due to the diarrhoea, and after stopping to take a breather on the draining board of a nearby sink, Gerald finally managed to throw the towel over him.

Still somehow managing to maintain his gentlemanly composure, Gerald handed the securely wrapped towel containing a very tired Eric over to me without saying a word and conducted the rest of the consultation in silence. I unwrapped different parts of Eric so that he could be fully examined.

The smell in the room was overpowering, my eyes were watering, and my ears were still ringing from Eric's screaming, but I held on until the task was complete.

Briskly and businessman-like, despite being heavily splattered with monkey faeces, Gerald informed Eric's owner of his suspected diagnosis and subsequent treatment plan. Gerald handed Eric's owner a handful of paper towel to wipe herself down with, motioned for me to place Eric back in his carrier, and escorted them both back out to reception, making no reference at all to what had just taken place.

As soon as they left the consulting room I sprang into action. Grabbing a bucket of disinfectant and a cloth, I began to clean the walls and surfaces, throwing a window open in an attempt to rid the room of the cloying odour.

Ten minutes later, Gerald reappeared, freshly clad in a new tweed jacket and trousers and smelling strongly of aftershave. He walked over to the heavily soiled photograph of his wife and the Queen, picked it up and handed it to me.

"I think this needs a bit of a wipe," he said, and with that, turned smartly on his heel and walked away.

Visit Hubble and Hattie on the web:
www.hubbleandhattie.com • www.hubbleandhattie.blogspot.co.uk
Details of all books • Special offers • Newsletter • New book news

21

Jenny

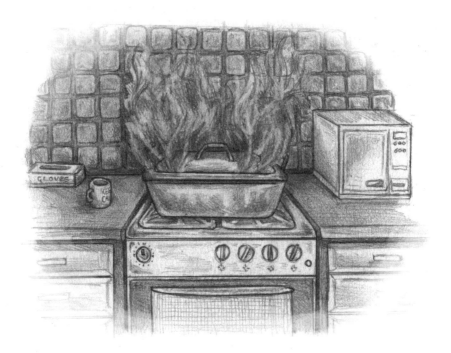

As well as the unconventional and delightfully eccentric Mr Crossland, another unforgettable character helped shape me into the veterinary nurse that I am today: our head nurse Jenny.

Jenny lived at the practice, in a small flat above the office. This often meant that Jenny's shifts rarely followed a set pattern. Jenny tended to be around most of the day in one capacity or another, and she devoted a lot of her own time to overseeing the care of any overnight patients. Jenny shared her flat with an ever-changing variety of different creatures. As well as her own two cats, Tigger and Bella (both ex-strays who had been handed in to the practice), Jenny's flat was also a temporary home for sick and injured wildlife, and occasionally she would also be asked to take in litters of orphaned kittens to hand rear. I became accustomed to seeing Jenny digging in the back garden, looking for worms to feed an injured wild bird, or being asked to mix up a batch of powdered milk at orphan kitten feeding time, and, of course, I always offered to lend a hand. Jenny was well known amongst local wildlife and cat charities, and was frequently called upon to help.

She was the archetypal matron who ran a tight ship, and I couldn't help but feel in awe of her as she threaded her way effortlessly through every working day. Jenny always had an accurate overview of where the vets were, including those out on farm and equine visits. She ensured that they were always equipped with everything they needed. She also kept a close eye on the reception team; she checked that consulting appointments flowed seamlessly, and that any emergency cases were dealt with in a timely manner.

Jenny really came into her own when working in the surgical unit, organising the daily operating lists, checking that the inpatients were properly cared for, and that they received their prescribed medications at the appropriate times. The care and attention Jenny gave to the animals in her supervision was exceptional: how I longed to possess the kind of animal handling skills that Jenny had. She was fearless, and exuded a confidence that put many a fractious patient at ease. I had known her to sit in a kennel for hours trying to soothe an anxious dog, and she had the ability to turn the most ferocious of cats into a cuddle-seeking, purring machine.

What Jenny had was patience, and she took the time to read her patients and understand what they needed to get the very best out of them. Whilst at the vets, most animals were completely out of their comfort zone, and needed constant reassurance that everything would be okay and that they were safe. Jenny always made sure that her patients were made to feel at ease during their stay.

Jenny was an efficient nurse, and seemed to be one step ahead of the vets when working through a hectic day of surgical procedures. The prep room and theatre would be scrubbed down and ready to go, and anaesthetic machines would be set up with the correct anaesthetic circuit matched to each patient. Sterilised packs of gowns, drapes, and instruments would be neatly laid out in preparation for each operation. Reels of suture materials would be opened and checked before use, and a dish of sterilised suture needles was freshly made up each day. Kidney dishes filled with skin disinfectant would be pre-prepared and lined up on a shelf in the prep room. Surgical clippers would be cleaned and oiled before each use. Breathing tubes (used to deliver fresh oxygen and anaesthetic agents via the anaesthetic machine once the patient had been safely anaesthetised by an intravenous induction agent) were laid out in the correct size order to match each patient. Jenny would also calculate the volume of injectable anaesthetic induction agent that each patient required, drawing it up into appropriately-sized syringes ready for the vet to check.

I loved to watch her work, and was fortunate enough to be able to shadow her during my first few weeks. Jenny taught me many of the practical skills that I still use today.

One of the most important things that Jenny taught me was the 'less is more' method of restraining patients. Most animals don't feel terribly at ease being handled by virtual strangers, and those feelings could be compounded if the animal was sick or in pain. By using gentle strokes, a soothing tone of voice, and employing your hands and body to steady the patient was always preferable to a more forceful approach.

Jenny also taught me how to make a 'cat pasty' when dealing with fractious cats if the aforementioned techniques failed. We dealt with a number of feral farm cats at the practice, who were not accustomed to being handled and often came in hissing, spitting, and lashing out with their claws. With the best will in the world, these feisty felines would never have succumbed to the charms of a 'cat whisperer,' not even one as talented as Jenny. This is where the art of cat-wrapping came into its own.

We kept a supply of large towels in a warm airing cupboard in the main building. When confronted with a non-compliant feline, a warm towel would be placed over them, covering them completely. The cat would usually put up a little resistance to this, but then allow themselves to be safely lifted from their carry basket or kennel. Cat and towel would then be placed directly on top of another warm towel that had been spread out on a table top. With considerable speed and dexterity, the towel on the table would be gathered up and wrapped snugly around the cat, securing their feet (including sharp claws) and their bodies, leaving only their heads poking out (for very aggressive cats sometimes the head was also included in the wrap). Once wrapped, the cat could be secured by the handler by tucking the cat into the side of their body with their arm. The warmth of the towel went some way toward soothing these cats, and the feeling of being securely covered also tended to help. The vet could then lift different sections of the towel to look at different parts of the cat's body. Once a full examination and treatment had been completed, the cat, still wrapped, could be safely returned to their carrier or kennel and the towel removed.

Jenny had many other tricks like this up her sleeve, and was always more than happy to share her knowledge with students, whether training to be a nurse or a vet.

As Jenny's working days and hours didn't really fit into any sort of shift pattern, we were all used to seeing her pop up throughout the day. I did, however, notice that she tended to disappear to her flat, around lunchtime most days, often not returning for an hour or more. No one seemed to be unduly worried about this, as Jenny would appear first thing in the morning and was usually still around at the end of the day, no matter what shift she had been scheduled to work. This midday break seemed to suit Jenny, because whenever she came back from an extended break, she always seemed to have a renewed vigour about her, tackling cleaning jobs with lightning speed, efficiently completing afternoon ward rounds with the duty vet, and ensuring that the day patients were all ready to go home. Jenny would also be a lot chattier during the afternoons, and I soon got into the habit of waiting until the afternoon to ask questions regarding non-urgent matters.

I assumed that Jenny was not a morning person, as her morning moods could be a complete contrast to her afternoon ones. Some mornings, Jenny would barely utter a word to her fellow colleagues; she would keep her head down and plough through her tasks in a moody silence. At those times, it was advisable to leave Jenny to her own devices, which is pretty much what everyone else seemed to do.

I was very naïve back then, and it wasn't until a few years later that I discovered the reason for Jenny's extended lunch breaks and her sometimes erratic and changeable behaviour. Jenny, it seemed, had a fondness for alcohol, and her afternoon breaks enabled her to enjoy the odd glass of wine. It did explain why she would emerge from her flat in the afternoon with a flushed face, smelling strongly of mint from the mouthwash she obviously used to disguise the alcohol on her breath.

I was reliably informed that Gerald Crossland was fully aware of Jenny's problem, but had never tackled it face to face. It was never really spoken about, and was never referred to by anyone who worked at the practice.

The one thing that I can hand on heart say, is that it never affected Jenny's abilities as a nurse when it came to patient care, and I guess at the time, that was all that mattered.

There were some issues that arose as a direct result of Jenny's afternoon wine-tasting sessions, and I got used to tackling these. The main problem we had was trying to prevent Jenny from burning the practice down – a dramatic statement perhaps, but a truthful one.

We had an old gas oven in the back kitchen, and its main function was to heat the autoclave that sat on the hob.

The gas burners on the hob were also used to sterilise some of the larger pieces of surgical equipment used by the large animal and equine vets. Some of these fearsome-looking instruments were just too big to fit inside the drum of the autoclave, and had to be sterilised using a different method.

To do this, we used an old-fashioned fish kettle – a long, rectangular, lidded enamel tray. The inside of the tray would be lined with a thick layer of cotton wool, the instrument that required sterilising would be laid on top, and a second layer of cotton wool placed on top of that. More cotton wool was packed down the sides, and a jug full of water poured in, enough to thoroughly soak the cotton wool. The fish kettle was then lifted onto the hob, and the two gas burners underneath it were lit. The instrument inside the fish kettle was steam-sterilised over a period of about an hour. The trick was not to allow the cotton wool to completely dry out, otherwise it would burn.

Jenny was always more than happy to set up the fish kettle, but if she did so just before leaving for one of her 'little breaks,' as she called them, she would often forget that she had done it. The first time I saw wisps of smoke drifting up the corridor from the back kitchen, I flew into a complete panic, rushing at top speed to be confronted by the alarming sight of smoke billowing out from under the lid of the fish kettle, along with the acrid smell of burning cotton wool. Turning off the gas burners, I used a tea towel to lift the hot lid of the fish kettle. The cotton wool had completely dried out, and the edges had started to blacken and char. I grabbed the nearest thing to hand, a mug of half-drunk tea, and threw its contents inside the fish kettle. With a hiss and a belch of steam, the would-be inferno was extinguished. With a deep sigh of relief, I continued to add water to the fish kettle until the cotton wool was once more soaked through.

I never did pluck up the courage to tell Jenny about her near miss, or, in fact, any of the near misses that we had by using this particular method of instrument sterilisation. We did, however, instigate a policy of always having a jug full of water in the kitchen every time we used the fish kettle. Jenny must have known that her colleagues covered up for her occasional misdemeanours, as she would sometimes come down to the kitchen and witness us trying to flap the smoke and steam out of the open back door with tea-towels, but she would simply walk by without saying a word.

These days, Health and Safety would have a field day with our antiquated ways of instrument sterilisation, but back then we just treated such things as part of the daily routine, and we learned to be extra vigilant and always prepared for the unexpected.

Visit Hubble and Hattie on the web:
www.hubbleandhattie.com • www.hubbleandhattie.blogspot.co.uk
Details of all books • Special offers • Newsletter • New book news

Scratching the surface

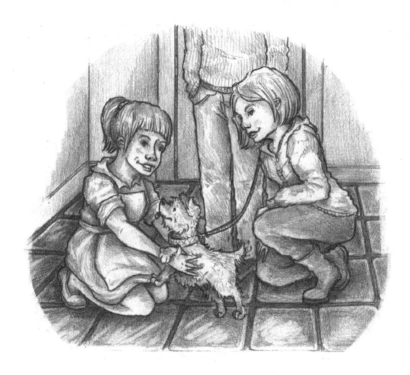

As my training progressed, my little green training book began to fill up as various tasks were signed off. I added copious notes to the book about the practical aspects of my day-to-day job. I found that the knowledge I was gaining from my studies at home, together with what I learnt at college, was constantly being put to practical use.

As with every aspect of my job, I usually started with the basics, and gradually worked my way up to the more complicated elements of different tasks, always listening to my peers, and always following instructions to the letter.

Some areas I genuinely struggled with, and laboratory work became a particular nemesis of mine. Most veterinary practices back then did not have an extensive range of laboratory equipment, with most of the lab work centring around the practice microscope and the preparation of slides of blood, urine, hair, or even faeces for microscopic examination. I could never quite get the hang of the steady-handed sweep of one microscope slide against another to create a perfect blood smear for microscopy, or the ability to prepare a slide for bacteriological examination without coating myself, my clothing, and most of the surrounding area with the bright red and blue stains required to highlight different cell types. I did, however, develop a talent for performing worm egg counts on faecal samples. These tests were routinely requested by livestock owners to enable them to make decisions on frequency of worming, or to check that their current worming protocols were effective. I quickly learned that this newly-acquired skill was not something to brag about. It was bad enough when word got out that I was completing this element of my training, because suddenly I became the recipient of dozens of containers of faeces from horses, cattle, sheep, and even the occasional goat. Lifting the lid on a tightly-sealed container of manure is not for the faint-hearted, particularly on a warm day when the aforementioned container has been sunning itself on a window ledge in the lab for a few hours. The containers ranged from the official plastic screw-top sample pots, which came with a useful little scoop in the lid, to re-purposed margarine or ice cream tubs. It didn't matter what size the container, you could guarantee it was filled to the brim. When trying to prise open the lid of an old margarine or ice cream tub, it wasn't long before I was automatically turning my head slightly to avoid the splatter that inevitably burst forth.

Laboratory work may have been messy, smelly and very exacting, but there was always a huge amount of satisfaction when you found something diagnostic whilst peering down the eyepiece of a microscope.

Tiny skin mites such as demodectic or sarcoptic mange, capable of causing immense discomfort to affected dogs when present in sufficient numbers, were commonly diagnosed via microscopy. The classic cigar shape of the demodectic mange mite was a complete contrast to the squat, round body of the sarcoptic mange mite, but identifying either one of these mites microscopically, and correlating the findings against clinical symptoms, meant that the correct treatment could then be administered. Nowadays, mange mite treatments are very straightforward, most cases responding well to either regular applications of a spot-on treatment or even a flavoured tablet given at prescribed intervals. Step back twenty plus years, however, and there was only one licensed treatment available, which came in the form of a strong-smelling chemical wash that had to be applied weekly. In most cases, dogs had to be thoroughly shampooed before the first wash was applied, and it was also advisable to have long-haired dogs clipped for the duration of treatment. The foul-smelling liquid had to be diluted with water, sponged all over the affected dog's body and then left to air dry.

We frequently admitted dogs affected with mange as day patients, to apply the wash ourselves, as some owners struggled to cope with the process. It was a relatively common sight to see a vet and nurse at the bottom of the garden sporting gloves and disposable aprons, with a trusty bucket at their side, sponging a patient from nose to tail. The smell of the liquid was so potent it was always a task that needed to be done outside in the fresh air whenever possible.

It was always worth the hard work and effort, especially when the cases were severe. And there's one case that always springs to mind: Harry, a little terrier cross.

Harry was found by a young couple whilst they were out on a walk one day. They spotted him lying curled up under a hedge by the side of a path. They were shocked by what they saw when they stopped to take a closer look. The little dog had no fur to speak of, just the odd tuft here and there, poking through his chronically thickened and damaged skin; skin that had grown almost like elephant hide. The dog's entire body was covered in painful, weeping, open sores. Feebly, Harry tried to lift a back leg to scratch himself, to relieve some of the intense irritation that he was feeling, but he just didn't have the strength. He had, it seemed, all but given up.

The couple, Ken and Lydia, didn't hesitate: they scooped him up, wrapped him in a picnic blanket they had in their car, and drove him straight to Greenfields, where Matthew, one of the duty vets, was waiting for them.

As soon as they arrived, Matthew whisked them into a consulting room, and I joined them, having heard that a very poorly dog had just been rushed in.

The first thing that hit me was the smell of the wrapped-up bundle on the consulting room table. The smell of chronically damaged, infected skin is unpleasantly musty, and tends to linger in your nostrils.

Matthew unwrapped the blanket and we caught a first glimpse of our patient, who was in a very sorry state indeed. Harry looked back at us, barely able to open his eyes due to the crusty scabs that were weighing down his eyelids, but he acknowledged our presence with a little wag of his stumpy tail. That tiny gesture told us all that we needed to know: there was a spark deep inside this little soul, a little flicker of life still there, and as we all know, every life is precious.

That tail wag strengthened our resolve to help; to give this dog a chance.

It wasn't just us who noticed the spark. Ken and Lydia, who had never owned a dog and never even considered owning a dog, offered to take Harry home to care for him and to administer any treatments that we recommended. Something about the plight of this poor neglected soul had touched their hearts, and they were only too willing to volunteer their help.

Suddenly, things were looking a lot more positive for this little dog.

Matthew gave him a thorough check over, and, despite every part of his body being incredibly sore, the dog allowed Matthew to examine his eyes, ears, tummy, chest, and heart. After checking his teeth, Matthew informed Ken and Lydia that Harry was likely to be quite young; no more than two years of age he thought.

The next step was to confirm what we thought was the underlying cause of hiss skin problem - demodectic mange.

Gently, Matthew took some scrapes from Harry's skin and smeared them onto several microscope slides. I took them straight up to the lab room, and popped the first one under the microscope. I wasn't in the least bit surprised to find a number of demodectic mange mites.

Demodectic mites occur naturally in dog hair follicles, but in certain circumstances, where the dog's immune system has been impaired, or if the dog is suffering from malnutrition, the mites can reproduce at a rapid rate. Subsequent skin damage can then allow secondary skin infections to take hold and, in some instances, severe cases of demodectic mange have proved fatal.

There was no way of telling for certain how Harry had got into such a state. Our best guess was that he had simply been abandoned by his previous owners.

But that was all in the past. Now, we needed to focus on the future, and begin the process of healing.

Together with Ken and Lydia, we devised a treatment plan. We kept Harry at Greenfields to enable us to start the course of chemical washes that would rid him of his troublesome mites. We also needed to assess his general health, and work out a feeding guide so he could start building up his weight, as he was extremely underweight. We were also obliged to report him to the authorities as a stray in case there was an owner actively looking for him (something we very much doubted).

As he turned to leave, Ken reached out to stroke him and murmured softly, "Harry. We will call him Harry. I think it will suit him. We'll see you soon then, young chap."

"Let's get to work," said Matthew. "You bring Harry and I'll get what we need."

Within a few minutes, we had assembled our wash station at the bottom of the garden and were ready to start.

First, we used a medicated shampoo, which we gently massaged into Harry's damaged skin to try to break down some of the crusts and grease. Although in quite a weakened state, Harry was able to stand, with just a little support from my steadying hand underneath his chest. Once the shampoo had been rinsed off, we began to apply the wash that would hopefully kill off Harry's mites and start to ease his discomfort. Harry's feet were badly affected, all four were very swollen and sore, so we stood him in a plastic litter tray and poured in some wash, to allow it to thoroughly soak in.

As the wash was designed to be left on and not rinsed away, once we were satisfied that Harry had been completely coated, I carried him into the surgical unit, and found him a kennel and a soft bed, where he could rest and dry off. Although obviously tired from his bathing session, Harry still managed a wag of his tail as he circled a couple of times before curling up in the warmth of his new bed. I watched for a while as he slept, hoping that Harry understood that he was now amongst friends.

Harry's subsequent recovery was little short of miraculous. After just over three weeks at Greenfields, we felt confident enough to hand the care of Harry over to Ken and Lydia. Harry really was coming on in leaps and bounds: this little dog who had all but given up on himself grew brighter and stronger every day. Through carefully monitored feeding, Harry was now getting the nutrition he so badly needed to help him on his road to recovery.

It was lovely to be greeted by Harry each day. He quickly fell into his routine of an early morning potter around the garden, followed by a small breakfast and his first dose of an antibiotic that was helping to clear up his badly infected skin. Harry couldn't walk far initially as he tired quickly, so we took it easy and let Harry tell us when he'd had enough and wanted to go back inside. But even after only a couple of days, Harry started to take more notice of his surroundings, pausing to stop and sniff or raise his nose in the air to catch a new scent. Elevenses followed breakfast, along with his daily vet check. Lunchtime always came with another short meander around the garden, and afternoon tea was always eagerly anticipated. Tea time brought with it a second dose of antibiotic and another small meal, and a bedtime treat was always delivered before Harry settled for the night. The little-and-often feeding regime is by far the best way to restore nutrition to those who have been denied it for long periods of time.

Over the next few weeks, Ken and Lydia brought Harry back for his weekly washes, and each time we could see the changes in him. His thickened skin started to soften, and the crusty scabs that covered his entire body began to fall away, revealing healthy skin underneath. New shafts of hair began to push their way through his healing skin, and bit by bit Harry started to look like a dog again. Before each bath, we took a few skin scrapes, and were delighted to see the number of mites reducing each time we examined them under the microscope.

Ken and Lydia were devoted to Harry. Diligently, they had followed our feeding instructions to the letter, and had been gradually building up his exercise. They had bought him a smart new collar and lead, and a vast array of different toys for Harry to play with. Harry slept at the foot of their bed each night in a huge padded dog bed; he even had his own blanket to cover him as he slept.

Once Harry's skin scrapes revealed no further evidence of mites for three consecutive weeks, we stopped the chemical washes and signed him off. Harry was now able to continue his new life free from pain and discomfort. This little dog had well and truly landed on his feet.

I bumped into Harry several months later, when Ken and Lydia popped in with Harry to weigh him. I could hardly believe he was the same dog! Gone was the smelly, mange-ridden bag of bones I once knew. The little dog jumping up around my legs, issuing little yips of excitement, with a stumpy tail that just didn't stop wagging, was bursting with health and vitality. I sank my fingers into Harry's newly regrown fur, revelling in its soft texture. Gone were the crusts, scabs and sores, and in their place a dense, full coat of brilliant white fur, but for a single brown patch over Harry's left eye. Harry danced and skipped around my feet as Ken and Lydia looked on, immense pride on their faces.

"Harry is such a character." Lydia smiled. "Everyone in our village loves him."

"I can see why." I laughed, scooping Harry into my arms, allowing him to smother my face with enthusiastic licks.

"We can't imagine life without him," said Ken. "He really does brighten our day. How anyone could have treated him so badly is totally beyond us."

I buried my face in the silky fur around Harry's neck, inhaling the scent of fresh shampoo, and whispered one word into his ear. One word that, for me, has so many different meanings: 'saved.'

Visit Hubble and Hattie on the web:
www.hubbleandhattie.com • www.hubbleandhattie.blogspot.co.uk
Details of all books • Special offers • Newsletter • New book news

A stitch in time

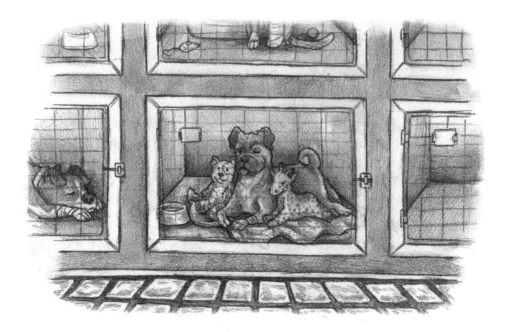

It was my first Saturday working as the only nurse in the practice. I had been at Greenfields for four months, and was feeling fairly confident about all I had learnt so far. Between the practical hands-on day-to-day experience, my days at college, and studying at home, I felt that I was making good progress, and was more than ready to take on some additional responsibilities.

I was not completely alone. I was working alongside Sarah and our Saturday vet, who, on this occasion, was James.

As there were no overnight inpatients, I had spent my morning in reception, helping Sarah with a bit of filing, and catching up with one or two cleaning jobs of my own.

Once the morning consultation session had finished, James left the practice following a visit request from one of our local farm clients. The weekend vet had to be a bit of a jack of all trades, able to deal with all aspects of work which included both small and large animals.

James left us with the telephone number of the farm he was visiting and went on his way. He was scheduled to return in time for the afternoon consultation session.

After cleaning and restocking the consulting room that James had used,

32

I set about making a cup of tea for Sarah and myself. I had only been away from reception for a few minutes when I heard Sarah call my name. I heard the degree of urgency in her voice, and quickly made my way back out to reception to find Sarah comforting a young girl. A woman, the girl's mother, was holding a bundled-up towel in her arms.

"It's Samson," she cried. "He's had a really bad accident."

I knew Samson: a cheeky little fawn pug who was always getting himself into trouble. A month or so earlier, he had managed to swallow a baby's dummy which subsequently became firmly lodged in his intestines, necessitating a surgical procedure to remove it. Before that, Samson had sustained a nasty cut to his back after getting caught on barbed wire when chasing rabbits whilst out on a walk.

"I don't know how it happened." Samson's owner sobbed, cuddling the towel bundle close to her chest. I could only assume that Samson was somewhere inside the towel she was holding on to so tightly.

"Samson was playing out in the garden with our friend's dog, Millie, when all of sudden we heard a yelp, and he came running in like this. I didn't know what to do – I just picked him up and brought him straight here."

"It's okay, Mrs Spencer, hand the little chap over and I will have a look," I said, with as much reassurance as I could muster.

Mrs Spencer thrust the bundle into my arms.

"I can't look," she cried. "I just know he is very badly hurt."

Carefully, I peeled away the towel to reveal Samson. I have to say, I could scarcely hold back a gasp of horror at what I saw.

Samson's left eye had popped clean out of its socket, and was currently resting on his cheek. His eyelids had clamped tightly shut behind it, preventing the eyeball from being returned to its normal position. Because it was still attached to muscle and the optic nerve, the eyeball wasn't dangling as such, it was just clearly not where it should have been. The eye itself, although looking quite gruesome, didn't appear to have been damaged, which gave me a glimmer of hope.

Pugs and similar short-nosed breeds are brachycephalic, meaning that their skulls are short and wide, giving these types of dog a very distinctive pushed-in face. Brachycephalic breeds like pugs also tend to have shallow eye sockets, which make them more prone to suffer from the condition exophthalmos (an abnormal protrusion of the eyeball), which could be traumatic in origin: for example colliding with another dog during play, which is what I suspected might have happened to Samson.

Samson recognised me straight away and I could feel his little corkscrew tail thumping against my side as I held him close. He looked up at me forlornly with his one good eye, and tried to nuzzle into the side of my neck, whining as he did so, obviously in a great deal of discomfort. I noticed that Samson had not travelled alone; snuggled up alongside him were his favourite toys – a very dog-eared giraffe and a badly chewed teddy bear – which always accompanied him on his frequent visits to us. These were Samson's comforters and went everywhere with him.

My brain rapidly fired into action as I mentally formulated a first aid plan for my patient, drawing on what I had learnt so far, both at work and through my studies.

"Right then, young man," I said, trying to instil as much confidence into my voice as possible. "We need to get you sorted out pretty sharpish, don't we?"

I asked Sarah to get in touch with James and tell him to return to the practice as quickly as possible.

I then spoke calmly to Samson's owner, Mrs Spencer, assuring her that I would attend to Samson straight away, and that we would do our best to save his eye.

Mrs Spencer gave me a grateful smile. "I know you will do your best for Samson. He does get himself into so much trouble." She leant forward and deposited a kiss on the top of his head, which was just about visible from within the towel he was swaddled in. "Now be a good boy, won't you, Samson?" Mrs Spencer put her arm around her daughter and led her out of the practice.

Holding Samson and his travelling companions securely in my arms, I took him to the surgical unit and popped him, together with his towel and friends, into a clean kennel, whilst I gathered any equipment I thought I might need.

The priority for Samson was to preserve the health of his eyeball until James was able to administer a general anaesthetic and attempt to place it back into its socket. Eyes are constantly lubricated by tears, and eyelids provide an effective barrier against injury. The longer Samson's eyeball remained where it was, the higher the chance it would become dry and damaged – potentially irreparably so.

I grabbed a bag of intravenous fluids containing a solution of sterile saline, a handful of large syringes, hypodermic needles, and a packet of sterile surgical swabs. I filled each of the syringes with saline solution. I used the first syringe to soak the swabs I'd put in a clean kidney dish, and placed the remaining syringes on the table in the prep room.

I collected Samson from his kennel. He was still very subdued and hadn't moved from inside the confines of his towel which was a good thing: the less he moved, the less likely he was to damage his eyeball.

I sat myself down on a chair in the prep room and placed Samson and his fluffy friends on my lap.

Gently moving the towel away from Samson's face, I picked up my first loaded syringe and slowly depressed the plunger, allowing a gentle stream of saline solution to flood over Samson's eyeball. I had to get the balance just right: if I was too vigorous, I feared I might damage the eyeball, but I also needed to exert enough flushing force to dislodge any debris that may have accumulated on the surface. Samson flinched a little as the cool fluid hit his face, but otherwise he sat perfectly still. Once confident that I had cleaned the eyeball as effectively as I could, I picked up some of the saline soaked swabs and very gently wrapped them around it. This would ensure that the eye stayed moist. Holding the swab-wrapped eye gingerly in one hand, I used my free hand to pick up another of the pre-loaded syringes and slowly dripped more saline onto the swabs. Now, it was vital that the swabs themselves did not start to dry out - if they did, they could adhere to Samson's eyeball. I also kepy a mental note of Samson's bital signs: his heart rate, respiratory rate, and his gum colour, all of which were fairly stable. Throughout the procedure, I used a soothing tone of voice, letting Samson know he was being incredibly brave, and that help was on its way.

Sarah came to say that James was on his way, but it still seemed like an eternity before I heard the door to the surgical unit being thrown open by James.

"Sorry I took so long," he gasped, trying to catch his breath. "What's been happening?" I gave James a brief summary, detailing the first aid measures I had taken.

"Great job," said James. After washing his hands, James gently peeled away one of the swabs to have a look at the eyeball underneath.

"Hmm, it doesn't look like the eyeball itself has been damaged, and well done you for keeping it from drying out. I think if we try to pop it back and suture Samson's eyelids shut for a time, we might just be able to save it."

Without further ado, James set to work, and within a few minutes, Samson had been anaesthetised, his eyeball flushed one more time, and with a little gentle persuasion, it was popped back into its socket. Once safely where it should be, James sutured Samson's eyelids together to ensure that his eyeball stayed put for the foreseeable future.

I remained with Samson whilst he recovered, having placed his giraffe and teddy either side of him so he knew that he was amongst friends. Listening to Samson's rhythmic snoring almost made me nod off too, as I watched the steady rise and fall of his chest with each rumbling exhalation. Eventually, Samson began to stir, he lifted his head groggily and fixed his one good eye on me with an unwavering stare.

I leant over to whisper in his ear: "it's going to be okay, Samson."

Samson returned the sentiment by giving my cheek a big slobbery lick before settling back down again into a snore-filled slumber.

It was two weeks before I saw Samson again. After an uneventful recovery, Samson had been discharged, with strict instructions to keep him rested.

Despite everything that had happened, including his previous visits for various other misdemeanours, Samson always bounced into the waiting room for his check-ups with boundless enthusiasm. Maybe because he knew there was a long queue of adoring fans all waiting for one of his extra special neck nuzzles.

Wearing a very fetching, Elizabethan, protective collar, and with one eye still firmly closed (giving a distinct impression that he was permanently winking), Samson bowled his way over to me, his whole body wriggling with excitement.

I scooped him into my arms for a cuddle.

"How has Samson been?" I managed to ask his owner whilst Samson covered my face liberally with licks.

"He has been marvellous," replied Mrs Spencer. "As good as gold. James is due to take his stitches out today. I am keeping everything crossed that all will be okay."

This was always a tense time. For two weeks, Samson's eyeball had been completely sealed off, hidden from view with no real way of telling how it was doing. Had we, with our speedy intervention, managed to save his sight?

I followed Mrs Spencer into the consulting room, and helped hold Samson on the examination table as, one by one, James removed the stitches.

Of course, giraffe and teddy were also in attendance, providing much needed moral support to their friend.

I could hardly contain my joy as Samson turned to look at me with two big, brown, beautiful, fully-functioning eyes. James confirmed that Samson's vision had been saved. I don't know who was happier: me, Mrs Spencer, or James. Maybe that honour went to Samson, who treated all three of us to yet another vigorous face wash. I like to think it was Samson's way of saying thank you.

Samson continued to be a frequent visitor to the practice, getting into one scrape or another, but it never dampened his enthusiasm. As far as Samson was concerned, as long as he had giraffe and teddy, things would always work out well in the end.

Dealing with Samson's eye was my first in a long line of emergency first aid cases, and one that I will never forget.

Visit Hubble and Hattie on the web:
www.hubbleandhattie.com • www.hubbleandhattie.blogspot.co.uk
Details of all books • Special offers • Newsletter • New book news

Calving capers

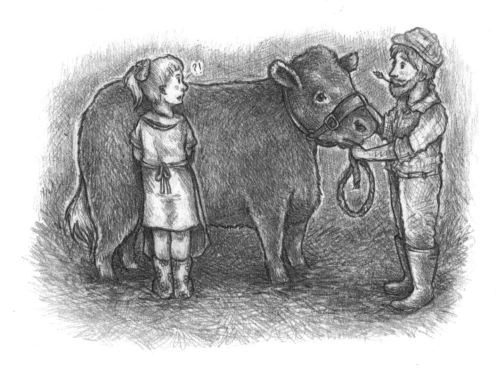

Greenfield Vets was a mixed small and large animal practice. The workload was pretty much evenly split between domestic family pets, horses, and farm animals. Over the years, the number of farms in the UK has reduced drastically in the UK, and, alongside general improvements in husbandry and animal management, this has led many vets to move completely away from the large animal sector. However, during my early training years, the large animal element of veterinary practice was still thriving.

I had a huge amount of respect for our local farmers, many of whom had been running their farms for generations. They were a hard-working bunch: honest, friendly, and, for the most part, quaintly old-fashioned. It was commonplace to see one of our local farmers at reception with 'shopping lists' of required medical supplies. In much the same way as vets tended to gravitate towards their universally accepted uniform of tweed and corduroy, local farmers could be readily identified by their heavy-duty work trousers – often splattered with all sorts of unmentionable things, with tatty bits of twine or lengths of frayed rope serving as belts – holey jumpers, and mud-encrusted wellington boots.

Farmers' shopping lists were often scribbled on old bits of cardboard, or on the back of used envelopes, and always presented us with the challenge of

37

deciphering the handwriting. Having to scrape off dried mud to see what was written underneath was the norm.

The nurses were often called upon to gather all the items on these lists, once the vets had checked and authorised their supply. This was a job I always liked doing, shutting myself in the large animal pharmacy, selecting the correct products from the shelves and ticking off the list as I went, filling a box with bandage material, tins of spray-on antibiotics (universally known as 'that purple spray'), tubs of powders that cured 'scour' (diarrhoea), and bottles of injectable antibiotics. I was always treated to a gracious nod and a polite thank you as they took their box of treasures and clomped out of the building, leaving a trail of muddy footprints in their wake.

Most of the time, the vets worked alone when they visited local farms and stables. The large animal vets would check the visit diary first thing each morning and divide the work between them. Gerald would always bag the equine work, leaving the other two large animal vets, Nathan and Gabriel to pick up the farm visits.

Nurses were rarely requested to assist with farm visits but when they were, there was no shortage of volunteers.

One morning, I was in the kitchen at the back of the practice, packing surgical kits, when Gabriel came to find me.

"Ah, there you are," he said. "I wondered if you fancied coming out with me tomorrow to Rowley's dairy farm? They have a cow booked for a planned caesarean as part of their dairy herd embryo transplant scheme."

Gabriel explained that the cow in question had been the recipient of an embryo transplant. That embryo had come from a larger and more expensive breed of cow, and it was predicted that due to the size of the calf, a normal birth would be unlikely. The calf's due date had been predicted, and the procedure booked in advance. The embryo transplant method was one way for dairy farmers to introduce different breeds of dairy cattle into their stock in a cost-effective way.

I agreed straight away and started to prepare a list of equipment that we would need to take with us on the visit.

The following morning, I was buzzing with excitement as we set off for Rowley's farm, armed with a boot full of equipment – which included a pair of wellington boots that I hadn't got around to replacing with a more sensibly coloured pair. These boots were a thing of beauty: bright pink and decorated with painted flowers in a riot of summer colours.

I also had a veterinary calving gown, which I'd managed to downsize to fit. These heavy-duty, waterproof, floor-length gowns, with elasticated sleeves at the top of each arm, were designed to protect the wearer from the elements as well as the less-than-savoury offerings from our generous farm-dwelling patients. I had tried on the smallest calving gown I could find at the practice, but was still completely swamped by it. However, with the skilful use of an industrial staple gun and a pair of scissors, I had managed to customise it to fit.

When we arrived at Rowley's, we were greeted by assorted members of the Rowley clan; a motley crew of strapping young men, headed by the patriarch of the family, known far and wide as Grandad. Dwarfed by his sons and grandson, Grandad spotted us immediately, took the length of straw he'd been chewing from his mouth, and used it to give us a welcoming wave.

The Rowley's were a well-organised bunch. They had cleared a small section of a barn for us and had lined it with bales of straw to form a little enclosure, inside which, our patient stood, lightly tethered to a wooden post. A bucket of soapy water and a towel were close by.

Ahead of our visit, a large area of fur had been clipped away from the expectant mother's hugely distended flank. After a final instrument check, and clad in our respective gowns and boots, Gabriel and I were ready to start.

Grandad positioned himself at the front end of the cow, took the tether in his hand and spoke gently to her as Gabriel injected her side with a local anaesthetic. Whilst this took effect, I prepared a kidney dish with a solution of skin disinfectant, and scrubbed the surgical site. We used the bucket of soapy water to wash our hands and uncovered arms, and shook them dry.

The Rowley boys sat on the bales of straw, watching expectantly.

I handed Gabriel a scalpel blade and he made a sweeping incision down the centre of the clipped and cleaned area. Using pre-sterilised cotton swabs, I dabbed at the wound edges, applying gentle pressure to staunch the bleeding from a small number of blood vessels that the scalpel had nicked. Surprisingly, caesarean sections are relatively bloodless. Once he had located and secured the cow's uterus, Gabriel made his second incision and began to lift the calf out. Following Gabriel's instructions, I held on to the incised edges of the uterus to stop it slipping back inside the cow while he gently manoeuvred the calf out. As soon as the calf was visible, the Rowley's jumped into action and gathered around us. I felt the heat that emanated from the calf as she was greeted by a cold rush of air. Two of the Rowleys stood either side of Gabriel, supporting the calf as she made her way into the world. With calm efficiency, they carried the calf away, set her down in a corner of the barn and began to rub her down briskly with handfuls of straw – this helped to encourage the newborn to take her first breaths. At the same time, the boys removed any traces of amniotic fluid from around the calf's nose and mouth so as not to obstruct its breathing.

Gabriel then started suturing the incision in the uterus.

I kept a hold on the uterus as Gabriel sutured, and I craned my neck to look over his shoulder to see how the calf was doing. Usually, by now, newborn calves, even those born by caesarean, would be starting to move, tiny hooves beginning to flail, and ears and tails starting to flick and twitch. But this calf was not moving; something was wrong.

"Gabriel," I whispered urgently. "The calf isn't moving. I don't think they're breathing."

Gabriel paused momentarily and turned to look.

"You're right," he answered. "That's not right at all, I'm going to have to intervene. Hang on to the uterus, it's going to start contracting. Don't let go, whatever you do."

With that, Gabriel set down his suture needle and stepped in to help the calf.

That left me and Grandad, who was still chattering away to the new mother, both seemingly unfazed by the drama unfolding around them.

As I could no longer see what was happening behind me, I concentrated on holding on to the edges of the cow's uterus.

After a minute or two, I realised that the uterus I was holding so carefully was, as Gabriel had warned, starting to shrink, and my hands were slowly being pulled deeper and deeper inside the cow. I shuffled forward a little and readjusted my grip, mindful that I was getting closer and closer to the side of the cow.

"Are you alright, young lady?" Grandad was looking at me, the same piece of straw that he had been chewing when we first arrived still clamped firmly between his teeth, bobbing up and down as he spoke. "You are getting a bit close to the old girl. Don't fall inside, will you?" He chuckled.

"I'll try not to," I thought, now up to my elbows inside the cow; the edges of the part-sutured uterus were still just about visible.

Behind me, there was a flurry of activity. As we suspected, the calf wasn't breathing, so Gabriel had instructed one of the Rowley boys to lift the calf by their hind legs and swing them back and forth, a classic method of ensuring that any fluid potentially trapped in the calf's airway, and causing an obstruction, was relieved. After the third swing, a cry went up, a sudden gush of fluid poured out of the calf's mouth and they started to breathe.

Things were not going so well for me …

Still desperately clinging to the slippery uterus, I was now up to my shoulders inside the cow, my face pressed against her flank. Cleaned and scrubbed surgical area aside, cows are not the most sanitary of beasts; I could feel my face being squashed into – what I could only guess to be – little dollops of cow manure ingrained in the cow's coarse coat. I was also being anointed with the stuff as the cow was now beginning to get quite restless, swishing her tail in an agitation. I had already been lashed several times.

"Grandad," I squeaked, finding it hard to move my mouth as it was squashed against the cow. "Grandad, would you mind giving Gabriel a shout for me? I'm getting a bit stuck here."

Grandad removed the stalk of straw from his mouth infuriatingly slowly, inspected it carefully, tucked it into his coat pocket, then called out to Gabriel.

"Here, lad, we could do with a bit of help."

Gabriel was back in an instant; after scrubbing his hands, he got straight back to work, completing the suturing in super quick time, much to the relief of my poor, overstretched arms.

By the time we had finished, the calf was already on her feet, tottering over to her mum, where she was instantly lavished with loving licks.

I gathered all the soiled instruments and set about packing everything away.

As I was walking back to the car, I passed Grandad, who was making his way back to the farmhouse. He beckoned me over.

"That was a good job well done, young lady," he said, pausing momentarily to extract the badly gnawed piece of straw from his pocket. He pointed the non-chewed end at me. "If I were you though, when you get home tonight, I would have a good soak in a hot bath. There is cow shit in your hair."

With that, he put the straw back in his mouth, burrowed his hands in his pockets, and wandered off.

I looked forlornly at my once-clean pink wellington boots, now coated with a layer of cow manure and mud, brushed the strands of manure-covered hair from my eyes, and shouted after him:

"All in a day's work!"

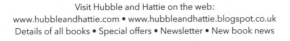

Visit Hubble and Hattie on the web:
www.hubbleandhattie.com • www.hubbleandhattie.blogspot.co.uk
Details of all books • Special offers • Newsletter • New book news

Breaking in and breaking out

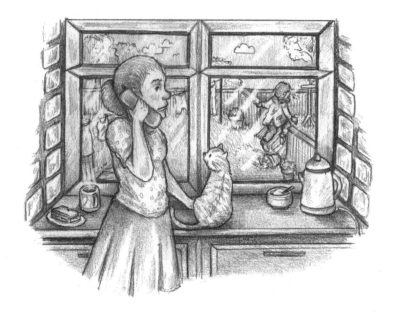

Diverse: another useful word when describing the role of a veterinary nurse. Every day a new challenge, every day a new adventure.

I loved the thrill of never knowing what was going to be asked of me, no matter how bizarre. Some of my most memorable tasks came via our local RSPCA inspector, Adam. Adam was a cheerful soul: with his cherubic apple-red cheeks and permanent smile, his visits to the practice were always welcome. On one occasion, he had a specific job for me.

"I need a housebreaker," he began, "and you would be the perfect candidate for the job."

Curiosity aroused, I couldn't wait to find out more.

A local resident had spotted (what they thought to be) a dog, all alone in a neighbour's house. They hadn't seen anyone return to the house for over 24 hours, and had also not seen the dog move from the sofa during that time. Concerned for their welfare, the resident had contacted the RSPCA, who duly followed up the call with a visit to the property.

"I have just been to the house and knocked on the door, but there is no one in," Adam explained. "I can see through the window, and there is, what looks like, quite an old dog lying on the sofa. Despite me banging on the door fairly loudly, the dog didn't respond at all. I need to make sure that they're okay. At the back of the property, there is a tiny window in the kitchen that's open. I need someone small enough to climb through and check that the dog is alright. Would you mind helping?"

Not needing to be asked twice, I checked with Jenny that it was okay to leave, grabbed my coat, and off we went.

The property was one of a long line of terraced houses in a nearby street, and as soon as Adam pulled up outside in his RSPCA van, a resident came out to greet us.

"Thank you so much for coming back. It's old Jim that I'm worried about." The neighbour explained that Jim, the dog, seemed to be alone, and no one had been seen leaving or entering the property for a good 24 hours. Jim's elderly owner, Edward, had also not been seen, which the neighbour felt most unusual as the two were usually inseparable. She, too, had spotted Jim seemingly asleep on the sofa, but had failed to rouse him despite repeatedly banging on the door.

All three of us made our way to the rear of the property, and Adam peered through the window before I did the same. We could see beyond the kitchen and into the lounge, where the large dog was lying motionless on the sofa.

"Hey, Jim!" I shouted, knocking on the window to get his attention, but there was no response.

I looked up and saw the small kitchen window, open just a crack. It couldn't open fully as there was a drainpipe in front of it, but maybe it was just enough for me to squeeze through. There was only one way to find out.

"Give me a bunk-up then, Adam."

Adam lifted me as high as he could, allowing me to grab hold of the windowsill and begin hoisting myself up and through. As small and slight as I am, it was a very tight squeeze, and when I was about halfway through the tiny gap, I nearly got wedged. With a nifty wriggle here and there, and some words of encouragement from Adam and the kindly neighbour, I got through.

I hadn't exactly planned my descent, so I landed, somewhat clumsily, head first in the kitchen sink, scattering an assortment of crockery and several of the potted plants that had been neatly lined up along the window ledge.

Flailing about wildly, I managed to climb from the sink and slithered to the floor. I looked straight towards the lounge area to see if the cacophony had disturbed the dog, but no, he hadn't moved.

I called his name as I slowly made my way into the lounge. Still nothing – no response at all from the motionless dog.

I admit, I was fearing the worst; maybe the old boy had passed away in his sleep.

Cautiously, I approached Jim and knelt by the sofa.

"Hey, Jim," I whispered, reaching out a hand to touch his head.

I nearly jumped out of my skin when Jim suddenly opened his eyes and fixed me with a curious look.

"Hello there, old chap. Have you been having a good sleep?" Jim responded to me gently rubbing the side of his ear, his tail thumping loudly against the sofa.

"You had us all a bit worried there," I continued in a low voice, so as not to scare him. After all, I was a stranger in his house, and I had obviously disturbed his restful sleep.

Jim didn't seem overly bothered about anything going on around him, and after emitting a big yawn, he slowly eased himself off the sofa and had a good shake.

The white flecks on his muzzle and the bluish tinge to the lenses of his eyes told me that Jim was indeed a dog who was in the autumn of his life. As handsome a dog as he was now, I could well imagine Jim was a real head-turner in his youth.

I watched as he ambled towards the kitchen, and followed him as he stood patiently by the back door.

The key was in the lock, so I opened it, and Jim pottered out into the garden.

"Is he okay?" asked Adam, his voice full of concern.

"He's fine," I replied. "I think the old chap may be a little hard of hearing, and he was so deeply asleep he just didn't hear a thing."

A smile of relief replaced the look of worry on Adam's face as he watched Jim wandering around the garden, not a care in the world.

"I wonder where Edward is?" said the neighbour. "It's not like him at all."

"I'll tell you what I will do," said Adam. "I'm free for the next couple of hours, so I will wait here with Jim to see if Edward comes back. Jim is obviously fine, but we do need to check that Edward returns soon, especially if this is out of character for him."

Adam called out to Jim, who, by now, had reached the top of the garden. Jim remained completely oblivious, sniffing at a nearby pile of leaves. I think this confirmed our suspicions: Jim was either completely deaf or severely hard of hearing. Upon realising this, Adam made his way to Jim and gently laid his hand on the back of his neck. Once again, the rhythmic swish of his tail indicated that Jim knew he was amongst friends, and he allowed Adam to guide him back into the house, where he promptly jumped back onto the sofa and settled down for another snooze.

And that's where we left them: Jim catching up with yet more beauty sleep, and Adam, armed with a dustpan and brush, sweeping up the mess I made when I fell through the window.

I walked the five-minute journey back to the practice and carried on with the rest of my shift.

Later that evening, Adam popped in to tell me that the mystery of Edward had been solved. Edward had been called away suddenly by a family emergency, and had left during the night, letting Jim out for his evening constitutional before he went. A friend had popped in briefly early the next morning to let Jim out and to give him his breakfast. Because the visit was so short, it had been missed by the neighbour, who was so used to seeing Edward and Jim at regular times throughout the day. Edward had set off to return home that day but got stuck in traffic, with no way to let anyone know. He was grateful to his neighbour for showing so much concern about his beloved dog, and confirmed that Jim was, to use Edward's own words, "deaf as a post," and could rarely be roused from a deep sleep.

With Jim and Edward happily reunited, Adam closed the case: I felt that, as a would-be cat burglar, I hadn't done too badly at all.

* * *

As far as breaking-in was concerned, it was a rarely utilised skill, but the opposite to breaking in is, of course, breaking out, an occurrence that was guaranteed to make veterinary professionals quake in their boots.

Working in veterinary practice you always have to be prepared to deal with the unexpected. No two days are ever the same: one minute you are contemplating whether or not to open the packet of biscuits you just found stashed somewhere, and the next you're haring down the road in pursuit of an escapee.

Just another ordinary day then?

When I started my afternoon reception shift one day, everything was ticking over nicely. Reports were that the vets were up to date with their farm visits, the morning appointment session had been straightforward, and the theatre list had been completed. There was an overall feeling of calm and order throughout the building.

The one sad note, as the early shift reception nurse, Liz, explained, was that a dog called Herbie had been brought in by his owners to be put to sleep. Herbie was a middle-aged lurcher who had become adept at escaping from his home and wreaking havoc in his local village. Herbie could open doors, climb out of windows, and had even managed to scale six-foot fences with ease.

Herbie's owners had tried their best to keep Herbie safely under lock and key, but a recent incident involving a flock of sheep had left them with the most difficult decision of all. They were so upset that they could not bear to stay whilst he was euthanised, and had bid him a tearful goodbye before leaving him in James' capable hands.

It was a very sad story, and my heart went out to Herbie and his owners.

When Liz finished her shift, I set about my first task of the afternoon – locating a pen. Pens were always a scarcity on reception, but after a time you got to know all the best hiding places. A feeling of smug satisfaction came over me when I opened one of the drawers under the reception desk: not only did a pen roll towards me, but following close behind, an unopened packet of chocolate biscuits. Jackpot!

I was just about to open the biscuits when the telephone rang. Reluctantly, I picked up the receiver.

At first, I couldn't understand what the caller was saying. There was a lot of garbled shouting, with a few expletives thrown every so often. A sense of incredulity soon set in as I started to piece together what she was trying to tell me.

She was, in fact, one of our neighbours. She had just looked out of her kitchen window and witnessed, to use her own words, "a great, big, hairy vet wearing a white coat vaulting over my garden fences." Sadly, the hurdling skills of this particular vet were reported to be very poor indeed, as he had knocked down several fence panels, including her own.

Naturally, she wanted an explanation as to why there was a vet rampaging through the local residents' gardens, leaving a trail of devastation in his wake.

Quite frankly, I hadn't a clue what was going on.

I apologised profusely and gave her my assurance that I would look into the matter immediately. I then agreed to send Mr Crossland around as soon as he returned from his farm visits, to survey the damage.

I left reception and made my way over to the surgical unit to see if I could find out what was happening. I was greeted by a sea of worried faces and there was no sign of James anywhere.

It seemed that James had walked Herbie into the prep room, and asked Jenny to assist him with putting Herbie to sleep. Jenny started to prepare the necessary equipment whilst James stayed with Herbie to provide him with some comforting strokes and tummy rubs.

Once everything was in place, James attempted to lift Herbie onto the prep table. At this point, Herbie seemed to sense all was not well, and suddenly jerked backwards, his collar slipping completely from around his neck. With lightning speed, he took off.

There were several doors between Herbie and the great outdoors that day, but each and every one had either been left slightly ajar, or was being opened by someone innocently passing through.

For Herbie, experienced escape artist that he was, negotiating his way through a few doors was a trifling matter. Within a few seconds, he was outside, making his way swiftly down to the bottom of the garden, with James following close behind.

Game on, as far as Herbie was concerned, as he squeezed himself through a tiny gap in the fence and into a neighbouring garden. James quickly worked out that he would not fit through the gap Herbie had found and decided that the best course of action was to try jumping the fence. It was apparent very soon that James' athletic skills were more than a little rusty.

Every time James got close, Herbie found another escape route. For the next hour, the two of them crossed several adjoining gardens. Herbie managed to traverse through each one effortlessly, whilst James, on the other hand, hit them all like a small hurricane.

We couldn't just stand by and leave James to single-handedly re-capture Herbie, so myself and Jenny volunteered to go out and help him. I arranged cover for reception and off we went in search of James and Herbie.

It wasn't difficult to pick up their trail – all we needed to do was follow the path of broken fence panels, trampled flowerbeds, and distraught local residents.

We eventually caught up with James in one of the neighbouring gardens, very wild-eyed and dishevelled. His once-white laboratory coat was now covered in mud and grass stains. His hair was a tangled mass of leaves, twigs, and general garden detritus.

As soon as he spotted us, James motioned for us to remain silent, pointing to a corner of the garden where Herbie was sniffing nonchalantly at a pile of leaves, seemingly oblivious to our presence.

With cat-like stealth, James slowly edged over to Herbie. Jenny and I held our breaths and crossed our fingers as James crouched down and stretched out an arm, desperately hoping that Herbie would lean over for a sniff.

Herbie did show a fleeting interest in James and rewarded his efforts with a brief lick of the hand, but then, with a flick of his fluffy tail, he disappeared through another convenient, Herbie-sized hole.

I could tell that James was not far off dissolving into a sobbing heap, so

I plucked some leaves out of his hair, brushed some dried clumps of mud off his coat, and instructed him to return to the practice whilst we continued to search for Herbie.

Dejected, James picked his way back over the wrecked gardens and left us to locate Herbie.

Between us, Jenny and I decided that hurdling fences wasn't really our style, so we opted for a more formal door-to-door approach, and set about asking the local residents to check their back gardens for our misplaced dog.

It seemed Herbie had simply vanished into thin air, and after knocking on many doors and drawing a blank each time, we returned to the practice empty-handed.

The telephones had been buzzing during our absence, and Lucy, who had volunteered to man the reception desk, had been fielding calls from irate neighbours complaining about the damage inflicted on their gardens by our roving vet. James was now ensconced in the office with a cup of strong, sugary tea, whilst he summoned the courage to make the very difficult call to Herbie's owners, informing them that their dog had absconded and we currently had no clue as to his current whereabouts.

As we were just about to start a busy evening surgery, Jenny and I returned to our posts, assuring James that we would resume the search later on that evening.

Our plans were brought forward when we received calls from concerned members of the public reporting that a dog matching Herbie's description had been spotted trotting down one of the side roads very close to the practice. Not wanting to miss the opportunity to catch him, Jenny and I set out once more. This time, we armed ourselves with some tasty treats and a slip lead, in the hope that if we could get close enough, we could tempt him then lasso him with the lead.

We headed in the general direction of reported sightings and when we rounded a corner, there was Herbie, about 500 yards ahead of us. He had stopped in front of an elderly couple who were leaning over Herbie, giving him a fuss. I started to shout at them, trying to get their attention, gesturing wildly at the lead I was carrying and pointing at Herbie, desperate for them to grab hold of him. They stood upright and waved cheerfully at me. Herbie gave me a cheeky backwards glance before casually lolloping off.

At this point, we broke into a run to catch up with him, but this proved futile: Herbie picked up speed and maintained his distance. He made a left turn at the end of the road, and by the time we reached the same junction, Herbie had disappeared once more.

We continued to look for Herbie, but there were no further sightings that evening. We eventually decided that we had no other choice but to abandon the search and resume the following morning.

I was on an early shift the following day, and as I arrived, I was just in time to see Jenny wheeling her pushbike out of the practice car park. She told me that Herbie had been spotted enjoying a game of football with a group of children on the local school playing fields. I wished her luck and she pedalled off at top speed towards the school.

I waited impatiently for news and she eventually returned, exhausted and alone. Herbie, she said, was in fine fettle, he had devoured a hearty breakfast of sandwiches and crisps, courtesy of the school children, and had taken up the position of midfield in a friendly kick-about. At half-time, Herbie left the playing field, making his way towards the local woods.

Herbie was really making the most of his liberation.

We sent out several search parties that day, and Herbie's owners had also recruited family and friends to help. They had taken the news of Herbie's escape very well, much to James' relief. After all, Herbie had devoted a lifetime perfecting the art of escapology, and had made it very clear that he wasn't quite ready to leave without one last adventure.

Over the next two days, I used every spare minute to go out and look for Herbie, either on foot or by car with James. I stopped everyone I met and gave them Herbie's description but to no avail: Herbie was still on the loose. I just prayed he was keeping himself safe.

On day three, we had a phone call reporting a Herbie-like dog wandering around a housing estate. After collecting the slip lead, I jumped into James' car alongside him and we headed off.

Within minutes, we arrived at the estate, and James slowly drove around, scouring front gardens and side roads.

I could scarcely believe my eyes when Herbie appeared beside us as we drove along. Looking no less worse for wear, Herbie cantered steadily alongside us as we drove: his fringed tail held aloft, waving like a flag, his mouth open wide, tongue lolling out to one side, looking for all the world like he was wearing the biggest grin

James wasn't sure what to do next, so he kept driving in the hope that he could somehow corral Herbie into an enclosed space. Ahead of us was a dead-end, so James dropped his speed and prepared to stop. This seemed to signal to Herbie that his game of chases was about to end, and he suddenly veered off to the side and trotted down a path.

By the time we had stopped and climbed out of the car, Herbie had once again vanished from sight and we returned to the practice once more, downhearted and minus Herbie.

Our luck finally changed on day four, when a call came through to say that a brown, rough-coated mongrel had appeared in a local resident's back garden. They had placed a bowl of chicken in their garage and managed to tempt the dog inside: the lure of a tasty bowl of food was just too much for Herbie to resist. He was finally safe.

James was quickly despatched, returning triumphantly a short time later with Herbie in tow.

James contacted Herbie's owners straight away, who were delighted to hear that their runaway dog had been recaptured. They said that Herbie's escapade had made them think long and hard about their decision to have him euthanised. Maybe, just maybe, with some additional training and a review of home security, Herbie's wanderlust could be curbed.

Herbie had a reprieve, and we all felt that we could finally breathe again.

When Herbie's owners came to collect him, we all gathered in the waiting room. There were multiple squeals of delight as we watched Herbie throw himself into one of his owners' open arms, smothering him in wet licks, tail thrashing wildly from side to side.

As Herbie left the building, flanked closely on either side by his owners, he did cast us one last backwards glance. He still wore that same wide-faced grin that he'd worn throughout his adventure, and to this day I remain totally convinced that he gave us a cheeky little wink, too.

Never underestimate the workings of the canine mind. Did Herbie know that his flight of freedom had been instrumental in saving his life? I'll let you decide.

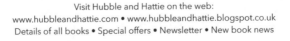

Visit Hubble and Hattie on the web:
www.hubbleandhattie.com • www.hubbleandhattie.blogspot.co.uk
Details of all books • Special offers • Newsletter • New book news

49

Happy as a pig in muck

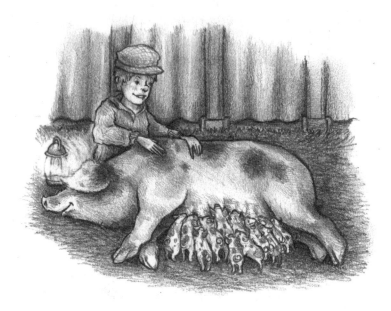

Another aspect of the job that made it so different from many other jobs, was the constant feeling of never quite being off duty. The vets at Greenfields shared an on-call night rota – there was someone available 24 hours a day, 365 days a year.

Jenny, being based on site, was often called upon at night, and was more than willing to help. There were no official arrangements for other nurses to be on-call, as a back-up for the vets, but every nurse I worked with at Greenfields always stepped up whenever they were asked to do so. There was always a little thrill of excitement when getting a call late at night or early in the morning.

I was once woken from a peaceful night's sleep by the phone ringing, a slightly breathless and panic-stricken Gabriel on the other end: "Sorry to bother you," he whispered (I wondered why he was whispering; did he think if he spoke any louder, he would wake the rest of the house?).

"I'm out at Carter's Farm, the owners are away overnight, and their son is taking care of the pigs. One of them is farrowing and there is a piglet stuck. I can't shift it at all and the only option is a caesarean to save both the sow and the piglets – any chance of help?"

There was an element of desperate pleading in Gabriel's voice along with a note of urgency. Of course, I agreed and told him I'd get there as soon as possible. Luckily, by this time, I'd passed my driving test and my parents had very generously bought me a car.

I dressed quickly and set off. It was just a little after one am, pitch black outside, with only a few glittering stars to light my way. After a quick stop at the practice to collect my bespoke calving gown and wellingtons, I made my way to Carter's farm.

As my tiny car bumped and rumbled along the track that led to the main house, I peered into the darkness, looking for signs of life. Suddenly, I spotted a little glow of light over by one of the barns, and after parking up, pulling on my boots, and grabbing my gown, I hurried over.

"I'm glad to see you," said Gabriel, a relieved smile breaking out on his face. "This is Tom." He indicated to the young boy standing next to him holding a battery-operated lamp aloft. "One of Tom's pigs, Bertha, has unexpectedly gone into labour, hasn't she, Tom?"

Tom nodded enthusiastically in response. "Bertha is my favourite pig, and a champion prize winner," said Tom proudly, straightening up and puffing out his chest. "She's a Gloucester Old Spot. Everybody loves Bertha."

"Bertha is having a little bit of bother: one of her piglets just doesn't seem to want to make an appearance at all, so we need to give Bertha a bit of a helping hand, don't we, Tom?"

Another vigorous nod from Tom made the lamp light bob up and down, reminding me of just how very dark it was.

"Most of the equipment I need is already in the pig shed where Bertha is," said Gabriel, pointing to the ground, where I could just about make out an untidy heap of instrument packs, swabs, needles, and cassettes of suture material. Gabriel had already filled a couple of additional buckets with soapy water.

"We just need to take this stuff over and then we can make a start." And with that, Gabriel grabbed one of his trusty buckets from the boot of his car, scooped up the instruments and other items from the floor. I offered to carry the equipment bucket whilst Gabriel took a water-filled bucket in each hand.

"Right then." Gabriel looked over at Tom. "Lead the way again, young sir."

Luckily, I had the foresight to put on my boots before even setting foot outside my car. The ground underfoot was quite wet, and as soon as we entered the field where the pigs were kept, I could feel myself sinking into the mud as I tried to negotiate through it.

Guided by the light from Tom's lamp, we picked our way across the muddy field. I couldn't see very much at all, other than the odd brick-built pig shed that suddenly loomed up out of the darkness. If I listened closely, I could hear the grunting, snuffling noises of the sleeping pigs surrounding us on all sides.

Eventually, we reached Bertha's shed, ducking our heads to pass through the low entrance, and pausing to wipe some of the mud off our boots on the straw-lined floor.

Our patient was lying on her side in one corner of the shed. One thing that always struck me about pigs was their sheer size, and Bertha, pregnancy aside, was gargantuan. She lifted her head to look at us as we entered, and gave a couple of quick grunts before letting her head drop back down to the ground. It was plain to see that Bertha was exhausted, with a belly full of piglets that needed to come out, one way or another.

The pig shed had no electricity, so we had no other light source than the lamp Tom was holding. I dragged a nearby bale of straw alongside Bertha and asked Tom to set the lamp on top of it. It wasn't ideal, but the halo of light that shone from it did provide us with some illumination at least.

Gabriel and I worked quietly and efficiently as we both donned disposable plastic aprons over our calving gowns. Gabriel drew up a large syringe of local anaesthetic, and assembled his instrument packs, scalpel blades, needles, and suture material whilst I scrubbed a large area of Bertha's flank. Tom perched on another nearby bale of straw, his eyes wide with anticipation.

"Right, here we go," announced Gabriel, as he made his primary incision into Bertha's side.

In next to no time, Gabriel had located Bertha's bulging uterus, and with a few deft movements of the scalpel blade, the first piglet appeared. Gabriel handed the squirming pink newborn over to me, quickly clearing the piglet's nose and mouth of fluid as he did so, and separated them from the placenta that had nourished them thus far. Grabbing a fistful of straw, I laid the piglet down and briskly rubbed them dry; the piglet kicked their legs and squealed in protest at the rude awakening. Vigorous rubbing of caesarean newborns helps to keep them warm and stimulates breathing. Thankfully, this little piglet needed very little help.

Caesareans for multiple births are incredibly fast-paced, and within moments, the next wriggling piglet was placed in my hands. Thick and fast they came: I stopped counting at eight, by which time I had recruited Tom to assist with the rubbing and drying process, a task he undertook with great care and diligence.

Eventually, we had a neat row of piglets, each one close against their brother or sister, so they could keep each other warm. The last piglet was in a breech position, and had effectively blocked the sow's birth canal. Unlike his siblings, this piglet wasn't moving at all; his skin had lost its healthy pink glow, and had a bluish tinge instead. Worryingly, the piglet also wasn't breathing. Gabriel cleared the piglet's nose and mouth of fluid and handed him over to me. I got to work straight away, rubbing at the piglet's chest with a handful of straw. I paused momentarily and placed my forefinger and thumb either side of his chest – sure enough, I felt the barely perceptible flutter of a tiny heartbeat.

"Come on, little fella," I murmured, as I continued to massage the piglet's chest, willing him to take a breath. I gave a huge sigh of relief when, suddenly, the piglet coughed, expelling a large amount of fluid, and kicked his legs furiously. I watched as the familiar healthy pink blush flooded across his body. Once he began taking regular breaths, I cleared a little space for him between his brothers and sisters and gently laid him down. Tom was made chief piglet watcher whilst I assisted Gabriel as he closed Bertha's wound. Time was of the essence, as we needed the piglets to start suckling from Bertha as quickly as possible, which, incidentally, became our next issue.

Newborn piglets are surprisingly mobile from birth, and these little ones were no exception. Out of the corner of my eye, I could see the once-neat line of piglets was rapidly becoming a jumble of tiny trotters and intertwined curly tails, as the newborns clambered over one another in search of their first meal. Tom tried his best to keep his miniature charges together, but as they all began to take their first few faltering steps, it soon became an impossible task. Responding to the soft grunts of their mother, the piglets began to make their way towards her.

As heart-warming as this was to observe, trying to prevent a gaggle of wobbly piglets from accidentally climbing back into Bertha's wound was a tad challenging. As fast as I removed one intrepid climber, another one took his place. Tom did his best, gently picking up each piglet and repositioning him or her in front of one of Bertha's swollen teats, expressing a little milk from each teat as he did so to encourage the piglets to start feeding. Within a few minutes, Tom had re-established control, and calm had once more descended inside the pig shed.

Now unhindered by clambering piglets, Gabriel quickly closed Bertha's wound. Fortunately for us, Bertha had been the model patient, and had thankfully barely moved an inch during the whole procedure. She now looked the picture of contentment with her new family alongside her. Tom had checked and counted all of the newborns and confirmed that there were twelve healthy piglets all now firmly latched onto Bertha, enjoying a much-needed feed.

Gabriel and I gathered our equipment back into the buckets.

"There you go, Tom," said Gabriel. "What do you think of that then? Twelve healthy piglets and a very happy Bertha."

"Smashing." Tom beamed, proudly looking over at his new family.

Once we had cleaned up, we sat for a short while on the straw bales whilst Gabriel explained to Tom that he would need to keep a close eye on Bertha and her piglets over the next few days. Tom would have to ensure that the piglets were being kept warm by their mum, and that they were all feeding regularly. Bertha would also need to have her wound checked daily to make sure that it was healing properly. Tom nodded solemnly as each instruction was given. Seeing the expression of intense concentration on Tom's face as he listened, told me that we were leaving Bertha in very capable (even if very young) hands.

"I think it's time to make a move," said Gabriel, gesturing to the lamp which was beginning to lose its once-bright glow. "I think the battery in your lamp is almost spent, Tom."

Without further ado, we gathered our buckets and bid a fond farewell to Bertha and her brood.

Outside, still in darkness, we made our way back across the field. As we walked, I had a distinct feeling that we were not alone. All the noise and activity coming from Bertha's shed must have disturbed her slumbering companions in the neighbouring sheds. The gentle snuffles and squeaks of the sleeping pigs had now been replaced by slightly more urgent grunts.

"If I were you, I wouldn't hang about," whispered Tom. "Some of these pigs can be a bit grumpy." With that, Tom broke into a steady trot.

We didn't need to be asked twice, and quickly followed suit, buckets swinging at our sides as we picked up our pace. My heart thumped as I heard what sounded like a large number of pigs rapidly closing in on us.

"Run!" shouted Tom, as he made an explosive dash for the end of the field, the light from his lamp perilously close to extinguishing, and plunging us into total darkness.

Ahead of me, I could just about make out the hedge that encircled the field, but because it was so dark, I couldn't work out where the gate was. There was nothing else for it: rather than be trampled underfoot by a horde of stampeding pigs, I threw my bucket over the hedge, gathered the bottom part of my calving gown, and attempted to follow the bucket. As I performed my death-defying leap, I felt a whoosh of air as another bucket sailed by, missing my head by inches. From the sound of rustling, and the snapping of twigs and branches nearby, I could only surmise that Gabriel had reached the same conclusion as me.

I have never claimed to possess any kind of gymnastic skills whatsoever, but I had somehow managed to vault over the hedge, despite wearing a cumbersome calving gown and a pair of heavy-duty wellington boots, all in the pitch black.

My landing definitely wasn't elegant, as there was a ditch on the other side of the hedge, and I ended up lying face down in a muddy puddle.

"Gabriel, are you okay?" I spluttered, spitting out a mouthful of brackish water.

A muffled groan came out of the darkness a few feet away, which at least confirmed that Gabriel was on the right side of the hedge.

Carefully, I got to my feet and stumbled towards the groaning.

"Tom," I called out. "Tom, where are you? We could really do with a bit of light."

"I'm here," replied Tom. The light he was carrying was now barely more than a pinprick, but it allowed a little illumination to fall on Gabriel.

I knelt next to him.

"Are we safe?" Gabriel uttered in a tremulous voice, fixing me with a startled look as he reached out to grab my hand.

The pigs had gathered on the other side of the hedge, and we could hear them snuffling and grunting in frustration that their quarry had managed to evade them.

I assured Gabriel that we were safe, telling him that we really needed to get moving before the lamplight gave up completely.

Gently, I helped Gabriel to his feet. He had twisted his ankle badly when he landed, so I asked Tom to support him whilst I tried to find all the equipment that now lay strewn about on the wet ground.

"Don't worry about your stuff," said Tom. "I will be over as soon as it gets light to check on Bertha. I'll have a good look around for anything that has been left behind."

Without further ado, I picked up the buckets and followed Tom and Gabriel as they made their way back to the farmhouse.

"Do you want a cup of tea?" Tom asked. "It won't take a minute to pop the kettle on."

One of the things that all farming communities had in common was their hospitality; no matter what the circumstances were, or what time of day or night it was, you could always rely on a steaming hot mug of tea to round things off.

Sitting in Tom's warm kitchen, I took a minute to study the many framed photographs that adorned the walls. Every single one of them featured a pig, and most also included Tom standing proudly next to his porcine pals, holding a rosette aloft. I recognised Bertha in several of them, too.

Knowing that not only had we more than likely saved Bertha's life, we had also saved the lives of her offspring, too, caused a warmth to spread through me, just as much as the hot, sweet tea, and as I looked across at the exhausted but contented face of Gabriel, I knew he felt the same way, too.

Visit Hubble and Hattie on the web:
www.hubbleandhattie.com • www.hubbleandhattie.blogspot.co.uk
Details of all books • Special offers • Newsletter • New book news

55

Jed's incredible journey

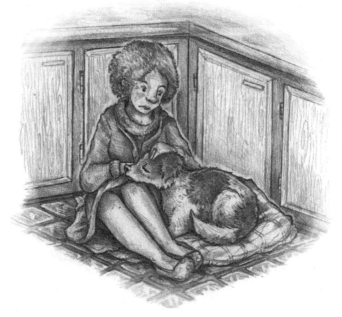

Apart from farm visits, vets are often called upon to make house visits, usually to euthanise elderly pets. Being able to say their final goodbyes in the comfort and familiarity of their own homes helps many owners come to terms with the loss of a beloved pet.

The memory of one particular house visit will always stay with me. Maybe not for the right reasons, but it reminds me that no matter what happens, you must always try to maintain dignity and professionalism, even when curve balls are being thrown at you, left, right, and centre.

We had received a phone call from a very distressed lady asking for a vet to come to her house to possibly euthanise her elderly dog, Jed, who had gone off his legs that morning. I packed the visit bag, mentally checking off the contents in my head, and set off to find the vet who was scheduled to attend the visit.

The duty vet that morning was a locum vet, William, who had only been at the practice a few days. William was a nice enough chap, though very serious, and liked things to be 'just so.' I found him studying a road map to confirm where we were going.

Once he spotted me, William folded the map neatly, and tucked it into his jacket pocket (tweed, of course).

I held up the visit bag to show we were ready to go, and minutes later we were on our way.

Conversation was a little stilted as we drove. Attending house visits for euthanasias were always a sombre affair, and I guess most of the time, both the vet and nurse were a little apprehensive about the task ahead. The weather matched our mood – grey clouds and persistent rain. I chose to focus on the hypnotic motion of the windscreen wipers as a distraction from the silence.

Following the map, we drove out into the countryside with very little around us other than sprawling open fields, interspersed now and again with farm buildings.

Eventually, we reached our destination: a pair of semi-detached houses set back from the main road. After checking the house name William had noted on a scrap of paper, he parked the car, climbed out, and knocked on the front door.

The door opened a crack, and tear-stained face peered out at us.

"Hello," said William, in a quiet but confident voice. "I am William, the vet, and this is my nurse, Tracey. We had a call today to say that Jed hasn't been well? Are you Mrs Roberts?"

"Please do come in," the lady replied, as she opened the door and ushered us inside. "My name is Angela. I am Mrs Roberts' neighbour. Barbara is terribly upset – it's just her and Jed you see, and he is so poorly. He can't stand up, and he's been very sick. I don't know if there is anything that you can do for him."

We followed Angela down a hallway and into a small, neat kitchen. In a corner, on top of a duvet, lay our patient, with his owner, Barbara, sat at his side, stroking his head.

"Hello old chap," said William, making his way over to Jed and kneeling on the floor next to him. I followed close behind, setting the visit bag on the kitchen table.

"Can you tell me what's being happening with Jed?" asked William, reaching out to give Jed a reassuring touch.

"It started a few days ago," replied Barbara, pausing to wipe a tear from her cheek. Barbara's red-rimmed eyes told of the worry and concern she was feeling for her beloved dog, and her voice trembled with emotion as she tried to choke back further tears.

"Jed has always had a good appetite," she began, "but he suddenly stopped eating. I can't tempt him with anything, even chicken which is his all-time favourite. Last night, he started being sick, and this morning he can't stand. He's been lying on his bed since I called you this morning. Jed is 17 years old, and has never had a day's illness in his life. I can't lose him. He is all that I have left since my husband passed away two years ago."

William placed his hand on Barbara's shoulder. "I'll have a look at him and see what we can do."

Jed didn't protest as William carried out his examination. A collie mix by the look of him, Jed's cloudy eyes and greying muzzle reflected his senior years. William started by lifting Jed's lips to check the colour of his gums. From where I was sat, I could see straight away that Jed's gums were deathly white instead of the normal, healthy salmon pink. Jed's tummy was also distended, and he winced a little as William gently palpated his abdomen.

After listening to Jed's heart and checking his temperature, William turned to Barbara.

"I'm afraid it's bad news," he said gently. "Jed has a large tumour on his spleen that has ruptured, causing him to bleed internally. He's very weak and is only going to get progressively more so. He's not in a great deal of pain at the moment – I think he just feels very tired."

Barbara sat up and took a deep breath. "I have to let him go, don't I?" she said, with a tremor in her voice.

"There is nothing I can do to save him," replied William. "The kindest thing that you can do for Jed is let us put him to sleep."

Barbara looked down at Jed, who had drifted off, his chin resting on her arm.

"I have to do what is right for Jed," she murmured, leaning over to kiss the top of his head.

We waited a short while to allow Barbara to say her goodbyes. It was important during these difficult times to allow owners time to say goodbye in whatever way they needed. I felt tears sting my own eyes as Barbara whispered to Jed that he would soon be reunited with his master who was waiting for him, where there were fields to run in and woods to explore. She thanked Jed for being such an important part of her life, and for all that they had shared together, telling him it was now time to say goodbye.

A brief nod from Barbara indicated that she was ready for us to help Jed on his final journey.

I had discreetly prepared all the necessary equipment, and William efficiently clipped a little fur away from Jed's front leg whilst I gently supported it for him. After a quick wipe with a swab soaked in a mild skin cleanser, William gestured to Barbara that he was about to inject Jed with an overdose of barbiturate which would allow him to pass away peacefully.

I don't think Jed was aware of anything other than being stroked and soothed by Barbara, who stayed at his side as he slipped away.

After listening to his chest with a stethoscope, William nodded to Barbara. "He's gone. Jed is at peace."

Barbara scooped Jed's lifeless body into her arms, buried her face into his soft fur and sobbed uncontrollably.

Barbara's neighbour, Angela, who had withdrawn to another room whilst we attended to Jed, returned, and gave Barbara a big hug. "You have done the right thing," she said.

We sat for a while longer to allow Barbara all the time she needed with Jed. After a little time, Angela gestured for us both to come away, so that she could speak to us.

In a lowered voice, Angela whispered, "I think Barbara knew in her heart that she was going to lose Jed today. Thank you both for what you have done for them – I know how hard it must be for you, too."

"That's perfectly okay," replied William. "It's what we are here for."

"We've spoken in the past about what Barbara wanted to happen with Jed once he had passed away, knowing that he was coming towards the end of his life," Angela continued. "And Barbara would like Jed to be buried, and I wonder, could you help?"

"Of course," said William. "What would you like us to do?"

"We have a close friend who is going to bury Jed for us. I have just called him, and he'll be able to bury Jed later this afternoon. Would you mind carrying him around to where our friend will be able to collect him? He's going to be buried alongside his brother, Bruce, in the garden of the house Barbara and her husband used to live in. Jed is quite a big dog, I won't be able to manage him by myself, and Barbara is in no fit state. If it's not too much of an ask ...?"

"No problem," said William. "I have a blanket in my car - we can wrap Jed in it, and Tracey and I will carry him wherever he needs to go."

I quickly popped out to the car to retrieve a large blanket - something the vets often kept several of in their cars for all sorts of different situations - whilst Angela explained to Barbara what we were going to do.

On my way back, I passed Barbara in the hallway. "I can't stay any longer," she sniffled, blowing her nose into a handkerchief. "I'm going to sit in my car until you've gone. Thank you both for being so kind."

"Not at all," I replied. "Jed was lucky to have had you as an owner. I can see how much he meant to you."

Barbara managed a weak smile before hurrying off outside.

I spread the blanket out next to Jed, and between us we gently lifted his body onto it and wrapped it around him.

In all honesty, lifting and carrying the body of the recently deceased is not the easiest thing to do. As Jed was quite a large dog, I can now fully appreciate where the expression 'dead weight' comes from. Nowadays, there are stretchers and robust body carriers with handles, but back in the day, it was a trusty blanket or bed sheet. We stood one at either end of Jed's carefully wrapped body - William at the head end, and me at the tail end. In unison, we each gathered our end of the blanket, lifted Jed, and attempted a slow and dignified walk towards the front door.

"No, no, no," cried Angela suddenly. "I can't have this. Barbara will be so upset to see Jed being carried out by two strangers." We stopped in our tracks whilst Angela stood to one side wringing her hands. Pausing, even for a moment, made me very mindful of just how heavy Jed was, and I had to readjust my grip on the blanket.

"I know," said Angela. "Could I stand between you and support Jed's middle as we walk past Barbara?"

William nodded in reply. Angela positioned herself between us and slipped her arms underneath Jed's body, supporting his weight from underneath, leaving myself and William with little to carry, but we continued to maintain our hold of the blanket at either end, and, albeit a little awkwardly, we manoeuvred ourselves outside.

It was still pouring with rain. I could see Barbara sitting in a car on the driveway, the windows a little misty. Barbara sat up and watched as we walked by, and I could just about make out the sound of a long, drawn-out wail coming from within.

Angela must have heard it, too, because when I turned momentarily I saw her face crumple, and with no prior warning, Angela let go of Jed, and buried her face in her hands, sobbing loudly.

What happened next was vaguely reminiscent of Cleopatra, in ancient Egyptian times, being rolled out of a carpet to present herself to Caesar. Poor

Jed rolled gracefully out of his blanket and onto the sodden ground in front of us, as well as his distraught owner.

A look of undisguised horror flashed across William's face. He still had his end of the blanket in his tightly clenched fist and I was still holding onto part of the blanket, too, standing momentarily frozen, rain trickling down the back of my neck, adding to the sudden chill I was feeling in my bones.

My ears were ringing with the anguished sounds coming from Angela and Barbara, who, by this time, had disappeared completely behind the misted windows of her car.

There was nothing else for it: stooping down, William and I lifted Jed, placed him back in the blanket, wrapped him up securely and tried again.

"Right," said William airily, giving Angela a waxy smile. "Shall we go?"

We carried Jed to the bottom of the drive, Angela tottering behind us, and we automatically turned into next-door's driveway. As this was the only property we could see anywhere nearby, we thought we were making a safe assumption.

"Where are you going?" trilled Angela.

"Is this not where we're taking Jed?" replied William.

"No, if you'd like to follow me, it's not far," was her response.

I was mystified. There was no other property in sight, but as we'd said we would transport Jed to his place of internment, we had no other choice but to follow Angela.

I don't know how far we walked down that particular country road; it felt like miles, and Jed seemed to gain weight with every step. The rain still hadn't let up, and the road was pitted with potholes and muddy puddles – I found a particularly bad one as I waded ankle-deep through it.

Still, we forged on, sloshing forwards with our precious cargo.

Eventually, I spotted a church steeple in the near distance. Surely that meant we were approaching a village or hamlet of some description. Eventually, Angela stopped in front of the church.

"Here we are."

"A church?" I said, incredulity in my voice.

"Yes, yes, come on through," said Angela, holding open the lychgate to allow us entry.

Could this get more bizarre? I thought, as we followed Angela through the graveyard towards the church itself. Angela led us to a large wooden door at the rear of the church.

"In here," she said, opening the door and ushering us inside.

We entered the church vestry, both of us, by now, feeling a little bemused.

Angela elaborated: "I rang Barbara's friend, our local vicar, whilst you were with Barbara and Jed. He's the one who lives Barbara's old house. He'll be here in a while to collect Jed's body to bury him in his garden. It's what Barbara wanted."

"Oh, I see," said William "so we just leave Jed here then?"

"Yes, please. I'll stay here with him until the vicar arrives. Can you find your own way back?"

We didn't need to be asked twice. We hurried out of the church and made our way back to the car.

Our return journey was mostly spent in subdued silence. We were both cold and soaked through. I glanced over at William, trying to gauge how he might be feeling about what had just happened. Initially, all I saw was a small, almost imperceptible twitch of his lips, which soon spread into a wide grin.

"Well," he laughed, slapping the top of the steering wheel. "Never let it be said that this job isn't without its challenges. Remember, it's how we rise to those challenges that makes us the people that we are."

I have never forgotten those wise words, and since that day, I've attended scores of house visits to euthanise pets and encountered many bizarre scenarios. I've helped dig numerous graves, attended many a burial ceremony, held a conversation with a stuffed dog (thinking it was the patient), and even had to be carried, fireman's-lift style, by a vet, down a treacherously icy path at one remote property during a particularly harsh winter. I have crawled under beds, become wedged behind sofas, and been accidentally locked inside a cupboard under the stairs.

I wanted a job that would always keep me on my toes, and that is exactly what I got.

Visit Hubble and Hattie on the web:
www.hubbleandhattie.com • www.hubbleandhattie.blogspot.co.uk
Details of all books • Special offers • Newsletter • New book news

High jinks

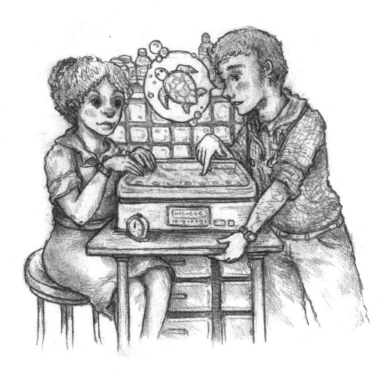

As my first year as a student came to an end, it was time to sit my first-year exams. Over the last 12 months, I had been studiously filling in my green training book and mastering an array of different skills: kennel cleaning, patient observation and restraint, inpatient care, and the dreaded laboratory work to name but a few. I had also been attending the weekly college lessons, and used my spare time to study my nurse training books. All of this was to culminate in a written exam, an oral exam, a practical exam.

As the number of trainee veterinary nurses was still quite small, there were a limited number of exam centres. The closest one to me, living in the Midlands, was The Royal Veterinary College in London. I didn't relish the prospect of travelling alone into the centre of London, but luckily for me, my lovely grandpa (who was immensely proud of the career path I had chosen) volunteered to arrange transport and keep me company. He neglected to tell me, however, that our chauffeur for the day was Stan, a one-legged, retired taxi driver who obviously fancied himself a contender for the next Grand Prix. I confess that I kept my eyes screwed tightly shut as Stan negotiated the busy streets of London at breakneck speed. Mind you, it did stop me worrying about the upcoming exam, as my primary concern was just getting there in one piece!

Eventually, we made it to The Royal Veterinary College, and I began to feel the fluttering of hundreds of tiny butterflies in my stomach as I gazed in awe at the magnificent building in front of me. Grandpa had already hopped out of the car and was digging in the boot for the bag with my outfit for the day - which was my first mistake.

I had spent the early hours of that morning contemplating the contents of my wardrobe, trying to figure out what I should wear. My uniform wasn't exactly pristine, and although it had progressed from the Victorian scullery maid look, it still hadn't quite caught up with the twentieth century. I had opted instead for neutrality by way of jeans and a jumper, but I'd picked up a spare lab coat from the practice as I thought this would lend a professional air during the oral and practical exams. Folding the lab coat over my arm, with Grandpa at my side, we walked through the double doors that led into the college.

We made our way over to the main reception desk. Out of the corner of my eye, I spotted a small group of student nurses deep in conversation. How did I know they were student nurses? Because they were all dressed in immaculate green-and-white pinstripe uniforms, with crisp white aprons, the tops of which bristled with pens, watches and other useful paraphernalia. I looked forlornly at the lab coat I had brought, and noticed several stains nestled amongst its many rumples and creases. A tangle of thread hung down from where a button once resided.

"Too late to do anything about it now," I mused aloud.

Grandpa reached the reception desk ahead of me. He stood politely to one side and waited for the receptionist to finish her phone call before stepping forward. He was usually such a softly-spoken man that I was startled by the sudden booming resonance of his voice, which seemed to echo throughout the building.

"This is my granddaughter," he announced loudly. "She is going to be a veterinary nurse." He followed this statement with a beatific smile, his blue eyes twinkling with pride.

I suddenly became very aware that the attention of everyone in the immediate vicinity was now fixed on us. Trying to hide, I sidled closer to Grandpa, and tried to tuck myself behind him. Noticing me there, he turned, enveloped me in a warm hug, and deposited a kiss on the top of my head. Squirming with embarrassment, I freed myself from his grasp and feigned interest in a pile of leaflets that sat on the reception desk.

The receptionist smiled at me, and I imagined that she probably had adoring grandparents, too, and knew exactly the pain I was feeling. She picked up a clipboard and ticked my name off a list. "If you'd like to join the others over there -" she gestured towards the group of students I had already noticed "- you will be called through for the written exam soon - good luck!"

"Now," said Grandpa, picking up my free hand and squeezing it tightly. "Do you want me to come with you? I'm sure they won't mind."

"That's very kind of you, Grandpa," I replied. "But I'll be okay, and I do think you should check on Stan."

After a hair ruffle and another large kiss, this time deposited on my cheek, Grandpa strode off, greeting everyone he passed with a chirpy hello and a cheery wave. I scurried over to the huddle of students and joined in with the general chatter until we were called through to sit the written exam.

I have to say that I like written exams. I enjoy pondering over questions and drawing on learnt knowledge to solve problems, and I couldn't believe how quickly the time had flown by as I answered the last question, set my pen down, and checked my watch.

Next was the oral exam. I felt quite apprehensive about this one, as I wasn't quite sure what to expect. I knocked on the oak-panelled door in front of me and waited until I was called in. I was greeted by four examiners seated at a long table. I sat directly in front of them, their warm smiles helping to calm my nerves.

As my first-year studies were mostly centred around anatomy and physiology (how different companion animals are made up and how their bodies function), the oral exam focused on topics such as the skeletal, muscular, and circulatory systems. I really felt in my comfort zone answering all the questions, and the examiners listened intently, taking the time to jot down notes as I spoke.

Before I knew it, my allotted time was up. I stood to leave and reverted to my old habit of adopting a half curtsey whilst walking slowly backwards, thanking the examiners for their time as I did so. Eventually, I ran out of floor and backed into a wall. Turning around, I found several identical doors, but which one was the exit? I could feel four sets of eyes boring into me as the examiners had already observed my strange backwards walk, and were now waiting to see what my next move was. There was nothing else for it: crossing my fingers, I grabbed the nearest door handle and flung open the door. The vacuum cleaner, mop and bucket, and array of cleaning products confirmed that I had, in fact, opened the door to a storage cupboard. My ears began to burn with embarrassment as I heard the barely perceptible sound of stifled giggles coming from behind me. I quickly closed the door and flashed the examiners an apologetic grin.

"I think the door on the far left is the one you want." One of the examiners pointed a pen in the direction of the correct door.

"Thank you," I squeaked gratefully and backed out of the room.

The rest of the day was spent on the practical exam, and I finally got the opportunity to don my lab coat for a while. I was asked to test a urine sample and record the results, and I had to peer down a microscope and identify a number of different parasites, as well as name the different types of cells in a pre-prepared blood smear. Again, I felt confident in the answers I gave.

The final test of the day was almost legendary amongst the nursing community – the 'spot test.' We were ushered into a classroom with several tables, all set out in rows. On the tables were various objects ranging from feeding bowls to brands of disinfectant to anatomical models. We were timed at each object and each came with an associated question. A series of paper arrows indicated the direction we had to move in, and each object was visited in turn, with never more than one student at each object at any time. A timer rang out to indicate when we had to move on.

There were two minor incidents during this part of the exam: a practical joker had moved some of the paper arrows, causing a bit of a traffic jam around one of the tables, which had to be quickly dispersed; and a fire bell rang out half way through the exam, which sounded very much like the timing bell that indicated when we needed to move on, leading to several students getting very confused and moving on too early.

I found the spot test to be the most enjoyable part of the day's exams, and I was especially pleased to see the urban legend amongst student nurses was, in fact, a reality. On one of the tables, floating in a bowl, there was what looked like a lump of clear jelly. The question: "what is this?" This seemingly harmless gelatinous blob was, in fact, a hydatid cyst that had been removed from a human being, and was the consequence of a tapeworm infection. I'd heard about this cyst from many of my peers, as it had been turning up at spot tests for years, stumping many of them.

As the final bell rang, signifying the end of the exam, I heaved a big sigh of relief. My feet were aching, and my brain was close to blowing a fuse, but I felt that it had all gone well: now it was a case of waiting to see if I had been successful, and if all my hard work and studies had paid off.

I headed off to find Grandpa, and was once more gathered into a bear-like hug. I was so tired that, luckily, I managed to sleep through most of the journey home, only jolted awake once or twice when some of Stan's driving manoeuvres didn't quite work out as planned.

It was several weeks before the results were issued. I remember my mum phoning me at work to say that a letter had arrived bearing the official stamp of The Royal College of Veterinary Surgeons.

My hands shook as I tore open the envelope that evening, and hastily scanned the contents within. I had passed! I was beyond ecstatic. I was halfway to realising my dream: one year successfully completed, one more to go.

I took my letter to work the following day to show my colleagues and we celebrated with cream cakes. After all, each and every one of them was instrumental in helping me achieve this first milestone.

I knew the good news had filtered back to Mr Crossland, but as it wasn't his way to communicate directly with his nursing staff, his congratulations came by way of a neatly typed letter – a letter that I still have today, carefully folded and kept inside my little green training book. A precious memory I will always treasure.

Year two of my training saw some changes at Greenfields. Although Jenny was still very much at the helm, we had said goodbye to Lucy, who was considered by us all to be Jenny's second-in-command, and the go-to person in Jenny's absence. Lucy had moved to pastures new, accepting a Head Nurse position at a large mixed practice in Yorkshire. This meant that I was given additional responsibilities, which included stock control, managing the nurses' rota, and helping with the training of new student nurses. The small animal side of the practice was growing all the time, and with it grew the nursing team.

I loved to see the fresh faces of new student nurses: They arrived wide-eyed and full of expectation, bubbling with excitement and enthusiasm. I was now feeling pretty much like an old hand at the job, more than ready to impart my knowledge and expertise to the next generation of veterinary nurses, and always felt a great sense of pride watching them blossom under my tutorage.

We always exposed our student nurses to the not-so-glamorous side of the job from day one. Just as I did, they started their induction with cleaning, cleaning, and yet more cleaning. We cheerfully parked them in front of sinks full of soiled drapes and instruments, and armed them with cloths, mops and buckets and got them scrubbing walls and floors.

There was also one very important initiation test that all our student nurses had to pass to secure their placements at the practice – the 'not keeling over in theatre' test.

We invited them into our operating theatre, usually on their first day, to observe some of the daily surgical procedures. Our theatre was quite small and always very warm. The combination of the heat, sights and smells had resulted in many wannabe veterinary nurses slumping to the floor in a dead faint. We knew that if one of us was spotted hauling a student out of the operating theatre by their feet, maybe the nursing career wasn't for them, and it was time for them to hang up their apron, so to speak.

For a long time, the one thing all students had in common was that they were all female: until the day I met Freddie.

Because of Mr Crossland's often lackadaisical and forgetful nature, we became adept at hiding the look of surprise on our faces when a potential new student nurse appeared in reception, and we always managed to maintain the pretence that we were fully expecting their arrival.

However, when I walked into the surgical unit early one Monday morning, I was taken aback by the sight of a lanky teenage boy – sporting a bristly moustache, clad in a vibrant t-shirt, and reeking of aftershave – warming his hands up under a wall heater.

"Hi," he said, reaching out to shake my hand. "I'm Freddie, this is my first day." In my haste to blurt out a reply, and attempt to disguise the fact I hadn't a clue who he was, I inhaled a little too deeply and suddenly found myself choking on the overpowering scent of his aftershave. As I coughed and spluttered, fighting for breath, tears coursing down my cheeks, I grabbed Freddie's hand and managed to croak a feeble hello and welcome. Looking slightly alarmed, Freddie let go of my hand and, without warning, slapped me firmly on the back between my shoulder blades.

"Thank you," I wheezed, giving Freddie a watery smile.

That's how it began: a friendship that has endured for well over 25 years. Freddie is still one of the quirkiest individuals I have ever had the pleasure of working with – funny, clever, kind, and compassionate, the kind of friend and colleague who will always be there for you through good times and bad. Freddie's teenage moustache matured with him over the years, and now and then, when the mood took him, he allowed it to blossom into a full, grizzly beard, much to the dismay of many theatre nurses, who were adamant that he should wear a surgical beard-guard mask (Freddie hated them). Freddie also never lost his fondness for smothering himself in aftershave. I just learned not to breathe too deeply after he'd applied a fresh coat.

Freddie was desperate to get on the veterinary nurse training course, and had recently completed an animal care course at a local branch of the RSPCA. As part of a government-funded training scheme, Freddie had been offered a temporary placement at Greenfields, three days a week. Never one to miss an opportunity, Mr Crossland requisitioned Freddie for the other two days, to work at his equine stud and stables that were about a half-hour drive from the practice.

Testimony to Freddie's determination, he accepted the offer and immediately set out to prove what an invaluable asset he would be if he were taken on as a full-time student nurse.

When he had to work at the stables, Freddie would cycle there and back, come rain or shine. He would spend the day mucking out stables and grooming horses before cycling back to join either myself or Jenny for the evening shift, unpaid and in his own time, purely to gain more experience. On the days he spent at Greenfields, Freddie threw himself into his work, often staying well beyond his normal shift times.

We weren't quite sure what Mr Crossland made of Freddie, and what he thought his role in the practice was. I received a scribbled note from him one morning saying that Freddie should be wearing a uniform whilst working in the practice, and that he'd found something suitable in his office.

Freddie went to look for his new uniform and appeared minutes later wearing a musty, brown stockman's coat that had clearly seen better days. After Freddie had spent a fortnight in the shabby garment, we could take no more, so we had a whip-round to buy him a new uniform: two pairs of smart black trousers, a green and white striped shirt, and a green v-neck sweater. I think this was our way of saying that Freddie was here to stay, and I shall never forget the look of pride on Freddie's face as he paraded up and down in his smart new uniform. Sadly, Freddie's catwalk-look did not last long: due to an unfortunate and unforeseen growth spurt, Freddie's trouser legs ended just above his ankles and we accidentally shrunk his sweater after putting it through a hot wash.

To this day, I am convinced that Mr Crossland was not involved in any decision-making regarding taking on Freddie as a full-time student nurse. Somehow, we managed to circumnavigate him, and it was a very special day for us all when Freddie brought in his shiny new green training book for the first time.

Another one of our most memorable students was Elaine. Elaine was also desperate to become a veterinary nurse, and put her heart and soul into every single task that was put her way. She passed the theatre test with flying colours, and attacked every cleaning job we gave her with vigour: our prep and theatre rooms gleamed.

Elaine took her role very seriously and followed every instruction to the letter; she really was a dream student, but her attention to detail and unwavering willingness to do exactly what she was told sometimes gave us the opportunity for a bit of light-hearted fun …

It had been a quiet morning. We'd finished all the daily procedures and Freddie had been dispatched to town to collect some medications from the chemist. After Elaine and I finished all the cleaning, I sent Elaine for her lunch break.

Freddie duly returned, having also popped into a sweet shop, bringing back many goodies, including a packet of mints, which he opened and offered to me. He stood for a while, contemplating the small, white, shiny sweets, before disappearing into theatre with them. A few minutes later he called me through and asked me to look in the incubator.

The incubator was our pride and joy. An ex-maternity hospital model, it had been donated by a grateful client, and was ideal for keeping small patients and neonates warm.

Freddie had carefully constructed a small, fluffy nest out of cotton wool, and placed several of the mints inside. He'd switched the incubator on, gently warming the mints as they nestled snugly in their new home. Freddie ushered me out, a mischievous smile playing on his lips.

Elaine returned from her lunch and Freddie told her that he had a very important job for her. Eager, she followed him into theatre and, side by side, they stood peering into the incubator.

Freddie explained that we had been given some turtle eggs to look after. The eggs were due to hatch imminently and it was vitally important that they were constantly supervised and the vet informed the minute they started to hatch out.

He pulled up a chair for Elaine, who sat herself down and did exactly what she had been told. She watched those mints intently, a look of total concentration etched on her face.

Freddie left her there for a good hour, popping his head around the door periodically to ask if there had been any changes. Elaine barely moved a muscle. In fact, I think she scarcely even blinked.

Eventually, Freddie decided it was time to call an end to his little prank and stepped back into theatre. He wandered casually over to the incubator, lifted the lid, plucked a mint from its comfy resting place, and popped it into his mouth.

I don't think I have ever witnessed such a change of facial expression as I did on Elaine that day. From focused intensity to abject shock, horror, and incredulity in the blink of an eye. A small strangled cry issued from her lips as she slid sideways off her chair. Freddie remained impassive and helped himself to another mint, licking his lips as he crunched his way through the crispy outer shell.

At this point, Freddie revealed, to a very startled Elaine, that she had, in fact, spent the last hour nursing half a packet of mints.

The tale of Elaine and the turtle eggs has to be ranked as one of the best student pranks ever, and never ceases to make me smile.

Despite the leg-pulling and the jokes, we were a close-knit team sharing a common bond: our need to 'fix' our patients, and nurture them back to full health. Being a job highly fuelled with emotion, it was also crucial that we learned to maintain a finely-tuned sense of humour. The ability to see the funny side of the most awkward of situations helped us through many a difficult day. Sharing that somewhat unusual (and, some may say, wholly inappropriate) sense of humour was another important factor in maintaining our close working relationships with one another. Remaining poker-faced whilst wrestling the urge to emit a hearty cackle was a skill I took pride in.

I found this particular facet of my personality of use one afternoon whilst engaged in one of my favourite pursuits: cleaning.

I had decided to give the prep room a proper spring clean, and had busied myself scrubbing floors and skirting boards, emptying out cupboards, and generally re-organising things. Jenny had given me an advanced warning that Mr Crossland was due to meet some clients later that afternoon and would be bringing them over to the prep room to view some X-rays.

Meanwhile, Freddie and Elaine were busy ministering to the tiniest of patients: a little hamster called Dave, who had developed pneumonia and was currently struggling to breathe. Despite James giving Dave's owners a grave prognosis, they had requested that we try to help him.

Freddie had set up an anaesthetic circuit to deliver pure oxygen to Dave, to see if it would improve his breathing. Whilst Elaine held a small length of tubing, connected to the anaesthetic machine, as close as she could to Dave's nose and mouth for a constant flow of oxygen, Freddie held his tiny charge in cupped hands to keep him warm. They were concentrating so hard on what they were doing, they scarcely seemed to notice Mr Crossland as he strode into the prep room with two of his best clients in tow. As they gathered around the X-ray viewer, Mr Crossland flashed me a benevolent smile. He liked nothing more than to show off his hard-working and caring team to a captive audience.

Sadly, Mr Crossland wasn't the only one who liked to indulge in a bit of show-boating.

Despite Freddie and Elaine's best efforts, poor Dave had passed away. However, noticing that the attention of Mr Crossland's guests was now firmly fixed on him, Freddie decided to give an impromptu demonstration of hamster resuscitation. Using the tip of his index finger, Freddie began to apply steady compressions to Dave's chest whilst barking out orders to a very bemused Elaine, instructing her to continue delivering fresh oxygen to his patient. The room fell silent. Everyone watched as Freddie battled valiantly with his tiny patient.

"We're losing him!" he cried. "Oxygen flush!"

As soon as I heard those words, a feeling of impending doom swept over me. Our anaesthetic machine had an oxygen flush button that released a burst of fresh oxygen, and the oxygen flush on this machine was well known for being a bit over-vigorous, and was to be used with extreme caution.

Fighting the overwhelming desire to screw my eyes tightly shut, I felt an almost toothache-like twinge of discomfort as Freddie held Dave in the palm of his hand, directly in front of the oxygen outlet pipe, and, with a flourish, pressed the oxygen flush button. The loud whoosh of air broke the pin-drop silence that fell again as Dave suddenly took flight, propelled by the force of the flushed oxygen.

Majestically, Dave soared past Mr Crossland and his cohorts before landing and sliding gently to a halt on top of the prep table in front of them. The look of undisguised horror on Mr Crossland's face was matched by his guests' and equalled by Freddie. Elaine's face had taken on a distinctly greenish hue and she looked as if she would pass out at any moment. There was nothing else for it: in a very matter-of-fact manner, I scooped up Dave in the cleaning cloth I'd been holding and walked nonchalantly away.

I've heard Freddie recount the tale, and what happened after I removed Dave from the scene, countless times:

The silence was eventually broken by a loud cough from Mr Crossland. "Right then, Mr and Mrs Green, as you can see from this X-ray, Tabitha's fracture is healing very well indeed. I should say that you'll be able to let her outside again within a month."

Still looking quite dumbfounded, Mr and Mrs Green looked obligingly at the X-ray that had been placed on the viewer, nodding in perfect unison.

Mr Crossland's cough had also, thankfully, stirred Freddie into action, and he gingerly started wheeling the anaesthetic machine out of the prep room. I think he was hoping to slip out unobtrusively, but due to a squeaky wheel, his departure did not go unnoticed and three pairs of eyes followed his every step.

Needless to say, Freddie's foray into the world of rodent resuscitation was followed up by a few choice words from Mr Crossland, and we were all encouraged to review our use of the oxygen flush button.

I could never help but chuckle when I heard Freddie tell the story to many a student nurse over the years, watching their eyes widen in awe as he described Dave's epic final flight.

Nothing, it would seem, would ever dampen Freddie's devilish sense of humour, and it wasn't long before he was back on top form again. One afternoon, I returned from a short trip into town, to see Elaine balanced precariously on the wall in front of the practice, staring intently at the roof.

"Everything okay, Elaine?" I asked.

"Yes, fine, thanks. I'm just waiting for the stork."

"Stork?" I replied, raising an eyebrow.

"Yes. Freddie has told me that we are expecting a visit from a stork. It's built a nest on top of the chimney. He asked me to wait here until it lands, and then to let him know straight away."

In all fairness, we did bring Elaine in before the rain got really bad, and Freddie did make her a consolatory cup of tea. Once she had eventually dried off, Elaine managed to see the funny side.

Freddie had a very agile mind, and was lightning quick when it came to spotting potential for a bit of fun.

Unpacking the daily pharmacy order from our supplier could sometimes be quite a mundane task. Ticking off all the different products against delivery notes, recording expiry dates, and placing the stock (in correct date order) in the pharmacy was a time-consuming process, but Freddie never missed an opportunity to inject a bit of humour into every aspect of his working day.

We were teaching a student, Marie, who was completing a two-week work experience secondment, about the varied role of the veterinary nurse. Most of the students we looked after were mainly interested in seeing what went on in the surgical unit, and if they didn't faint on their first foray into theatre, we always made sure that they saw the full extent of what we did. But our work wasn't always glamorous and exciting; we had our fair share of less interesting tasks to perform.

Marie was picking each item out of the boxes, checking them off against their corresponding delivery notes. To make this job a little more interesting, Freddie or I would explain what each product was and what it did. As we were a mixed practice, treating domestic pets as well as farm animals and horses, our daily deliveries were quite large, and contained a wide range of different products. There were bottles and bottles of injectable penicillin for sheep, cattle, and pigs; syringes of penicillin that could be administered directly into the teats of cattle to deal with conditions like mastitis; boxes of large animal stomach powder that treated a myriad of digestive system upsets; huge tins of ringworm treatment powder (something that we all grew to loathe, as we had to accurately measure this unpleasant-smelling powder into dozens and dozens of paper dispensing envelopes); rolls and packs of bandaging material; large tubs of tablets; and trays of vaccines, to name but a few. Each item had its own use in improving health and welfare, and provided the practice with an extensive armoury of products to combat sickness.

Marie had successfully emptied one box of products and had almost finished her second when she pulled something from the box, regarding it with a puzzled expression.

"What's this?" she enquired, holding the mystery item aloft.

The item in question was, in fact, completely irrelevant; it was merely the bottom off-cut from a large, clear, heavy-duty polythene bag. Approximately sixteen inches in length, it formed a shallow V-shape when straightened out. The boxes our deliveries came in often contained random bits of packaging – cardboard, scrunched up paper, bubble wrap, etc – and this happened to be one of them.

I was just about to explain this when Freddie, mind sharp as ever, got in first.

"Ahh," he cried, plucking the strip of polythene from Marie's hand. "I've been waiting for this to arrive. Would you like to guess what it is?"

Marie looked completely baffled (as did I), and shook her head.

What on earth was Freddie up to now, I wondered.

"This," said Freddie dramatically, "is a specially-designed snake bath."

I literally had to put my fist in my mouth to prevent the giggle from spilling out.

"Wow," said Marie in wonder. "How does it work?"

Freddie laid the length of polythene on top of a nearby table and lovingly smoothed it out.

"Here's what you do," he replied, earnestly. "You take this bath and fill it with a small amount of skin disinfectant that has been diluted with warm water, and then you pop the snake in lengthwise. Snakes love the feeling of the warm water and they won't move until you lift them out. Great for snakes that are having trouble shedding their skin."

"Gosh," said Marie. "That is totally awesome, I would love to see that."

Needless to say, we told Marie what the polythene actually was soon after, and once again Freddie was banished to the nurses' naughty step (or in our case, made to scrub the theatre floor with a toothbrush).

As for Marie? She finished college and went to study at university, qualifying as a veterinary surgeon several years later, so I guess we can chalk that one up as a success.

A star is born

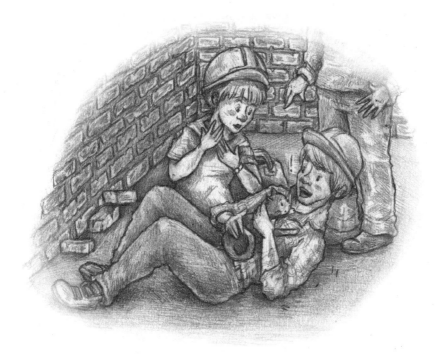

Dogs may have been the most common patients the small animal vets treated at Greenfields, but the number of feline patients brought to us was slowly starting to rise as their popularity as pets increased. During my early years as a veterinary nurse, I began to realise that a lot of cats lived a fairly 'latchkey' existence: let out in the morning and back in again at night. It was commonplace for many cats to be left out overnight, too. As time moved on, cats began to enjoy a more pampered lifestyle, being welcomed into the heart of many families.

Cats can be fiercely independent creatures, as most cat owners will happily tell you, which is one of the reasons they are now so popular as pets. Cats have a talent for self-sufficiency, which is well suited to today's busy world. Cats are also, essentially, prey animals, and as such, they are masters of all disguise when it comes to illness. If a cat is displaying signs of illness, then it really is feeling very poorly; cats do not play the sympathy card. It is simply not in their genetic make-up to do so.

The mantra drummed into every student vet and nurse, during training and beyond, is that cats are not just small dogs. They command an entirely different method of approach. This meant that cats could be some of the trickiest patients to treat, as they gave so few hints by way of clinical signs, often behaving quite normally until things reached a critical point. This did, however, mean that treating our feline friends brought many rewards – the most soul-enriching being the time you heard the first rumbling purr of a cat who was recovering from serious illness or injury.

Cats also possess their own unique armoury of self-defence, especially if they decide they don't like you and don't want your help. Not only do you have to be wary of their teeth, but they also have multiple sets of sharp, shiny claws that can be used with pinpoint accuracy.

Cats are also not open to bribery, unlike their canine counterparts. Offering a feline patient a tasty treat in exchange for compliance tended to elicit a haughty look of disdain, followed by a succession of rapid tail flicks: an early indicator that this method of approach was going to fail dismally.

Despite all of this, I was, and still am, a massive fan of cats, and have been lucky enough to share my life with some wonderful characters over the years. One such character was the imaginatively-named, Pusskins, a beautiful long-haired tortoiseshell, with more than a hint of Persian in her ancestry, who was rescued by me and my mum from a block of flats.

We received a call at Greenfields one morning to report that a feral cat had taken up residence in the lobby of a block of flats, and was apparently terrorising the occupants daily.

As the flats were only a few minutes' walk from my house, and I wasn't due to start work until the afternoon, Jenny telephoned to ask if I would go along and see if I could catch the cat. Mum offered her help, so armed with our hastily thrown together 'savage cat collection kit' (comprising two pairs of rubber gloves, large towels, and a cat basket), we walked down to the flats.

When we arrived, we were greeted by some of the residents, who cheerfully regaled us with tales of the savage beast who had taken to stalking them and jumping out when they least expected it. With Mum following close behind me, we cautiously entered the building, mindful that at any moment we could be under attack from the marauding moggy. We had both put on our rubber gloves – the best form of protection we could find at short notice – and I had the towel ready to throw over the cat to ensure a safe capture for all involved.

On tiptoe, we walked through the main reception area, looking for signs of life. The residents present had opted to remain outside whilst we conducted our search. I wondered how on earth we were going to tackle this fearsome creature once we had located them.

I didn't have to wonder for much longer, as we found our feral cat curled up under a flight of stairs, next to a heater.

Surely this couldn't be the same cat? The little scrap of fluff asleep in front of us was barely more than a kitten. Slowly, I knelt, removed my gloves, reached out a tentative hand, and stroked the cat gently on the back of her neck (I could safely say 'her' at this point because of her tortoiseshell markings, which are only present in female cats except in very rare cases). She woke instantly with a little squeaking meow, got up, and had a luxuriously long stretch, followed by a lazy, wide-mouthed yawn that showed her needle-sharp teeth, before regarding me with her glittering emerald green eyes.

She was a beautiful cat: semi-longhaired, her silken coat was a marbled mix of black, white, and ginger, with a huge set of whiskers that fanned out either side of her tiny pink nose. I looked around at Mum who was still poised, rubber-gloved hands at the ready, should our little vagabond decide to show her true colours.

"Are you the little hooligan we're looking for?" I murmured softly, using the back of my hand to rub the kitten under her chin. She responded by butting her head against my hand, and as she did so, I felt the rhythmic vibration of a soft purr. It was going well so far, so I reached over and carefully picked her up, bringing her close to my chest.

"Be careful," whispered Mum as I cuddled the kitten, speaking softly to her all the time. The purring didn't stop, even when I stood up and placed her in the cat basket we'd lined with one of the towels.

As we walked out of the block of flats, the residents looked at us in awe, scarcely able to believe that we had captured the furry little renegade.

We took home our little stray, and offered her some cooked chicken, which she devoured with relish. I sat and watched her as she ate, still a bit puzzled about how one so small and charming had been capable of causing so much trouble. After finishing her meal, the kitten washed her face with her paws before casually strolling up to me and jumping on my lap. As she snuggled up against me and closed her eyes, I felt a distinct tugging on my heartstrings.

"This little lady isn't going to go far," I mused. And she didn't. Pusskins, as we named her, was home.

Did this innocent little bundle of cuteness ever show the feisty side that had struck terror into the hearts of so many? Yes, she did!

Pusskins was what we, as veterinary professionals, called a 'naughty tortie': capable of an almost Jekyll-and-Hyde-like transformation, sweet and unassuming one moment, and a hissing, spitting ball of fire the next. Fiercely independent, Pusskins knew what she wanted and how to get it. We learned to be respectful of the twitching tail that could herald an accurately timed swipe of the paw, and we were always mindful of entering rooms in case she was behind the door, ready to pounce.

We had a rose arch in our back garden, which, during the spring, was covered in hundreds of tiny pink clematis flowers. Pusskins liked to sit on top of the arch and bury herself amongst the flowers. Pity the poor unassuming person who walked underneath the arch, as Pusskins would suddenly drop on top of them, whilst emitting an ear-shattering shriek, before leaping to the ground and running off at top speed.

Pusskins was indeed a naughty cat - free-spirited, adventurous, and brave - but we loved our little firecracker, and she taught me so much about cats, especially how adept they are at wrapping you around their soft little paws. When people say they own cats, I am quick to remind them that truthfully, it's the other way around: I have happily been owned by several cats over the years!

As well as being the masters of all disguise, cats also have an inherent love of exploring, coupled with a natural curiosity about the world around them. I'm sure that if you could meander through the complex maze of a cat's mind, you'd see the words 'I wonder if I could fit into that?' appear frequently.

confessions of a veterinary nurse

You only have to scroll through social media these days to find countless images of cats who have crammed themselves into all manner of different objects. Plenty of cats have been photographed squashed into plant pots, vases, handbags, and shoes, to name just a few examples. There is no doubt about it: cats just can't resist the magnetic pull of confined spaces and the overwhelming desire to check them out for size. And if they're not climbing into things, they're climbing up them, which is perfectly fine if the cat in question can climb back down again.

I recall spending a frantic cold winter's evening trying to encourage Pusskins down from a neighbour's roof. She had climbed onto the rooftop during a snowstorm, and by the time she'd decided to come down, everything was covered in a fresh blanket of snow. This meant that from Pusskins' perspective, everything now looked like it was on the same level. Usually, to get down from the roof, she'd hop onto the neighbours' shed roof before jumping down to the ground, but the snow was confusing her – she just couldn't work out where the once familiar shed roof was.

After hours of watching her pacing back and forth and listening to her plaintive cries, we asked our neighbours if they minded us clearing some snow from their shed roof. Once we had swept some snow from the roof, as well as a small patch from the ground beneath it, Pusskins climbed straight down, and we got a good telling off from her for leaving her up there for so long.

I resisted the urge to call the fire service to help Pusskins down from the roof, but some cat owners seem to have the fire brigade on speed dial. One such owner had a cat named Sam, who was a huge ginger tom cat and couldn't stay away from the big oak tree in his owner's back garden. Although possessing the skill and agility to climb the tree, Sam never quite got to grips with the downwards journey. Unable to cope with Sam's persistent wailing every time he got stuck in the tree, the fire brigade was frequently dispatched to retrieve him from one of his many leafy perches. Sam was never grateful to his saviours for plucking him to safety, and always rewarded them with a token scratch or two. In sheer desperation, Sam's owners resorted to having the tree cut down to prevent further incidents. All was well for a while until Sam discovered a neighbour's conifer, and the cycle began again.

The only time I have ever attended a cat rescue at the request of our local fire brigade was in response to a call that a cat had been discovered trapped between the exterior walls of two adjacent disused factory buildings. A local resident had contacted the RSPCA after hearing its distressed cries. Although not visible, the cat's persistent yowling had drawn the resident to the tiniest of gaps between the two buildings. Adam had been dispatched to help, and, by use of a powerful torch, had managed to roughly locate the cat. This was where things started to get complicated. Somehow, the cat had got wedged between the walls of the neighbouring buildings, and was trapped approximately three feet off the ground, several feet from where Adam was standing. No amount of cajoling or waving an opened tin of sardines at the entrance of the tiny gap could convince the cat to move, and Adam surmised that the poor cat was well and truly stuck.

The fire brigade was summoned to help, along with veterinary assistance from me and James. Adam wasn't sure how long the cat had been there, as the surrounding area was pretty much deserted, and it was just by chance that someone had been walking by and heard the cat's calls.

I wasn't quite sure what to pack, even as I checked the vet's visit bag before leaving. Syringes, needles, intravenous catheters, bandaging materials, and a bottle of sedative were amongst the things I thought might be of use. I noted that the bottle of sedative already in the bag had only a few drops left, so I added a fresh bottle, just in case. Armed with a cat basket and a couple of large towels, we set off.

Once we arrived at the scene, we were somewhat taken aback by the presence of a small crowd. The factories backed onto the local post office and it was pension day. The sight of a fire engine had piqued many a curious mind and the pension queue had redeployed itself. I saw Adam amongst the rapidly growing crowd and waved him over.

"I'm glad to see you guys," Adam said, his rosy-red cheeks slightly more flushed than usual. "If you can fight your way through the spectators, the fire crew guys are in there." He gestured towards one of the factory buildings, which was in a very poor state of repair indeed. Picking our way through the crowd - and over several piles of rubble from where parts of the building had collapsed - we joined members of the local fire crew inside. Adam introduced us to fireman Dan, who was leading the fire crew team. Dan gave me a bone-crushing handshake and a rather fetching hard hat that was way too big for me.

"Hi, guys," he said. "Thanks for coming. A bit of a tricky one here, and we're not quite sure how to proceed."

Dan explained that the cat seemed to be completely stuck between the two walls, and the only solution they could think of was to drill a section of the wall, as close to the cat as possible, and then ease him through the hole. Dan added that it could be risky: the wall was old and a little unstable, meaning it could collapse as soon as the drilling started. The other issue was that the cat's exact position was difficult to work out - the hole would have to be close enough to allow safe passage, but far enough away to avoid any accidental injury. None of us knew how long the cat had been trapped there, or if he had sustained any injuries. Between us, we agreed that this was the best, if not the only, option available to us.

By now, the crowd of people outside the factories had grown considerably. Adam went outside to move them back to a safe distance. A photographer from the local newspaper had also turned up, and was poised with his camera, ready for action.

I stood back and watched as Dan and his co-workers marked out a section of wall with chalk, and slowly started to drill into the brickwork. Brick dust filled the air as small chunks of the wall began to crumble and fall away.

"Gosh, the poor cat must be terrified," I murmured, turning to James. I did a quick double take - James was no longer standing next to me!

I peered outside and soon spotted him. In true British spirit, during times of crisis, you could always rely on someone to produce a teapot to make even the most desperate of situations seem just that little bit brighter. Perched on a nearby wall, along with several pensioners, James was dunking a chocolate biscuit into a steaming mug of tea that had been graciously supplied by the staff at the post office. Cheerily, James waved his half-eaten biscuit at me and shouted, "thought I would wait out here – health and safety you know." James paused mid-wave and beamed as the photographer snapped a quick picture of him.

This all seemed to bring out the hitherto unknown showman in James. Putting his mug on top of the wall and wiping the biscuit crumbs from his face with the back of his sleeve, James suddenly jumped up and addressed his captive audience, who were more than willing to hang on to his every word.

"Don't be alarmed everybody," he began. "The situation is perfectly under control. Our amazing boys in the fire brigade are going to create a hole in the wall from which I, James, the duty vet, will extract the poor trapped cat. Before we can attempt removal, I am going to administer this powerful sedative so that the cat doesn't get too distressed." With a theatrical flourish, James produced the bottle of sedative from his pocket, which he must have removed from the visit bag. As he did so, a shower of syringes and needles fell from his pocket. The crowd gasped as James held the bottle aloft. I groaned inwardly as I noticed that the bottle he was holding was the almost empty one, something I am sure the watching crowds were bound to notice. Quickly, I dug around in the visit bag, located the new bottle of sedative, and hurried over to James. As soon as he saw me, James obviously spotted the opportunity for another photo. He grabbed my arm, and stood me next to him, still holding up the bottle, and wearing a dazzling smile. By sleight of hand, I managed to grab the near-empty bottle and swap it for the full one, seconds before we were snapped on camera, James looking like a worldly, confident professional, me looking slightly flustered in my ridiculously over-sized hard hat.

"James, I think you are needed back inside," I said in a slightly pleading tone of voice, tugging on the sleeve of his coat. After helping him collect the objects that had fallen out of his pocket, I finally managed to shepherd James back into the building.

By this time, the fire crew had managed to drill a football-sized hole in the wall.

"I think that is as much of the wall as we can safely remove," explained Dan. "I've reached inside and I can just about touch the cat. I hope that it's enough."

James gently inserted his arm inside the hole and began to feel for the cat.

"Got him!" he exclaimed. "Well, a back leg at least."

The cat responded to James' touch by emitting a loud howl. James then tried to see if he could manoeuvre the cat towards the hole, but he just wouldn't budge – he was still jammed.

Withdrawing his arm, James stood back, deep in thought.

"What I think we need," he said, "is some sort of lubricant, to enable us to move the cat without causing injury." James went back outside and addressed the audience again: "can anyone get me a bottle of washing up liquid?"

Several hands went up, and a volunteer was dispatched to the corner shop, returning minutes later with a bottle of washing up liquid.

Whilst we waited, James drew up a small volume of sedative. We didn't know how heavy the cat was or his current state of health, so the dose had to be guessed rather than accurately calculated. Administering the sedative was James' next challenge. Having to rely on touch only, James put one hand back into the hole and relocated the cat. Once he had one hand on the cat, James reached in with the loaded syringe. There was a cry of protest from the cat as James somehow managed to inject the sedative.

"I don't exactly know where that went," said James, "but it's definitely in the cat."

After waiting several minutes for the sedative to take effect, and hopefully relax the cat, James set to work with the washing-up liquid. Making up a soapy solution with warm water (once again supplied from the post office), James soaped his hands and slowly began to soak the parts of the cat he could reach. Despite feeling a little drowsy, the cat started to meow furiously, not appreciating the warm, soapy liquid one bit.

The crowd outside fell silent, and you could almost feel a collective holding of breath as James slowly began to ease the cat towards the hole.

"He's coming," he whispered. "Get ready with the towel."

I'm not sure what happened next: I can only assume that the gap between the two walls widened as, like a cork from a bottle, James pulled the cat out of the hole, overbalanced, and fell backwards, clutching the cat to his chest.

Although sleepy, the cat was not feeling particularly grateful about being rescued, and wriggled and squirmed in James' arms as he struggled to keep a hold of him. Swiftly, I threw my towel over the cat and scooped him into my arms. Adam held open the lid of our cat basket, and I dropped the cat inside, bundled up in the towel, and secured the lid.

Throughout, I was mindful of the clicking of the photographer's camera, which had captured every moment of the heroic rescue.

I helped James to his feet and brushed off the worst of the brick dust that now covered him. Quickly regaining his composure, and not wanting to miss out on his five minutes of fame, James staggered outside and announced to his adoring new fans that the cat had been successfully rescued, and that his life had undoubtedly been saved.

A huge cheer went up from the crowds, and a rousing chorus of *For He's a Jolly Good Fellow* followed suit. I looked over at Adam and we treated each other to simultaneous eye rolls.

Time was now of the essence. The cat needed to be assessed for any injuries he might have sustained, and it was also important that we cleaned and dried him as soon as possible. The sedative, as much as it aided the rescue, would have decreased the cat's body temperature, and the soaking he got from the soapy water was likely to have caused a further drop, which could potentially become life-threatening.

After thanking Dan and the fire crew, we packed our equipment away, loaded the cat in the car, and made our way back to the practice. Adam followed in his van, keen to see how the cat fared.

Once back at the practice, we took the cat straight over to the surgical unit. Still completely covered by the towel, he was very quiet and not moving. James picked up a section of the towel and tentatively lifted it away. The cat, looking very bedraggled and forlorn, had curled itself into a tight ball. James gently picked him up and placed him on a fresh towel on the prep table. He didn't protest at all as we began to clean away the soap using warm water and a couple of clean cloths. As we cleaned, we checked for any obvious injuries, but apart from the odd graze and being a bit on the thin side, it seemed that he'd managed to escape serious injury. It was as we inspected him that we found he was male, only a youngster, jet black in colour, with four white paws and a white tip to his tail.

Once thoroughly cleaned, I gathered him in my arms and began to rub him dry. From deep within the towel I could just about make out the beginnings of a quiet purr. I unwrapped him a little bit and a soggy face with a droopy set of whiskers popped out.

"Hey there, little fella," I soothed, using a corner of the towel to rub under his chin. "I think someone is starting to feel a little better."

The cat responded with a series of chirping meows. Although still a little groggy from the sedative, he was becoming more alert, his rusty purr growing louder by the minute. He seemed to be almost enjoying himself as I continued to massage his body, ensuring that the last of the soapy suds were removed from his coat.

"I think someone might be ready for something to eat, too," I concluded, carrying him through to a clean kennel.

I wasn't wrong there. As I spooned a small amount of cat food into a dish, he rubbed himself back and forth against the front of his cage, pausing once or twice to stick one of his front paws through the bars as if gesturing for me to return.

I was scarcely able to set down the bowl inside the kennel, before he dived straight in and ate every scrap, looking up at me expectantly once he had finished, hoping for more.

"That's it for now, cheeky boy." I laughed, wiping a bit of cat food off his nose. Judging from his response, I guessed that he'd been trapped for some time. How he had come to be there in the first place was a mystery, but for now, he was safe, and was assured board and lodgings for as long as he needed them. Now, we needed a name for our little stray, even if it was just a temporary one.

Our town was historically linked to the hosiery industry, and as it was a wall of an old sock factory that we'd had to drill through, we christened him Sox.

We tried to find Sox's owner over the next couple of weeks. Jenny and I knocked on the doors of houses near the factories, and we also put a notice in the post office, but no one came forward to claim him. Sox was such a friendly cat, and so playful that he was rapidly becoming a major distraction for everyone, as no-one could resist stopping at his kennel to dangle a toy in front of him, watching as he stalked and pounced. Although he had a huge list of admirers, Sox had really worked his charms on Adam, who had taken to popping in after his day shift to see how he was doing. None of us were surprised when Adam admitted that he had well and truly fallen for Sox and wanted to adopt him.

It was a happy day for us all when we waved goodbye to Sox, purring away in his cat carrier, sporting a snazzy, glittery collar bearing a shiny new identity tag. A bag full of toys accompanied Sox as he went home with Adam and his family.

And was our heroic rescue mission recorded? A week after we had liberated Sox, James came rushing over to me, brandishing a copy of our local newspaper.

"Have you seen this?" he said excitedly.

Sure enough, we had made front-page news with our daring rescue. To this day, I'm unconvinced that the choice of photograph was wholly appropriate. The photographer had snapped the exact moment that James had fallen flat on his back, clutching Sox to his chest. He'd also caught the look of surprise on my face, as well as on the faces of several firemen.

"What do you think?" asked James proudly. "Have they got my best side?"

I took the paper in my hands and scrutinised the grainy image.

"I think," I replied, handing the paper back to him, "if you look closely enough, you can see that you have chocolate on your chin."

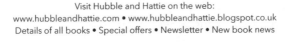

Visit Hubble and Hattie on the web:
www.hubbleandhattie.com • www.hubbleandhattie.blogspot.co.uk
Details of all books • Special offers • Newsletter • New book news

Throwing a lifeline

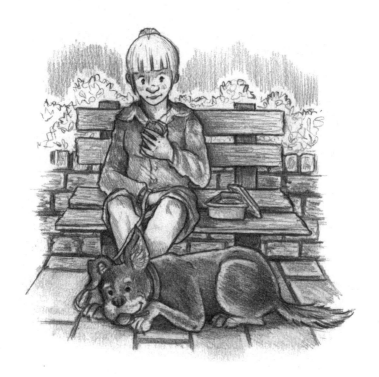

As most other practices did, Greenfields occasionally became a temporary refuge for waifs and strays. Jenny was often the first port of call for cats and wildlife, but she also indulged in a bit of dog rehoming from time to time.

Thankfully, the need for Jenny to step in and offer help to a dog who was otherwise facing a very uncertain future was a rarity, but when she did, grateful sighs of relief could be heard all around the practice.

The system whereby a dog owner signs their dog over to a local veterinary practice to rehome still exists today, but is very much bound by red tape, and maybe rightly so. It is a process that is undoubtedly best left to rescue centres.

Step back almost thirty years and such bureaucracy didn't exist. Rescue centres were smaller in number, with fewer intake spaces available. It was a dilemma that many practices faced: when a healthy dog was brought in for euthanasia, simply because the owner could no longer care for it.

What do you do? Veterinary professionals cannot refuse a direct request from an owner to euthanise a pet that belongs to them, but ending a healthy life doesn't rest easily on the conscience of any vet.

We were lucky: we had our canine guardian angel, Jenny.

When faced with the prospect of having to euthanise a healthy dog, the owners were asked if they'd be prepared to speak with Jenny before making a final decision, and thankfully most were more than willing to do so.

Jenny would then try to obtain some background on the dog – things such as temperament, medical history, and the reason why the decision to euthanise had been made.

If, after discussion, Jenny felt that the dog could potentially be rehomed, the owners would then be asked to officially sign the dog over.

To cover the dog's board and lodgings whilst they stayed at the practice, Jenny would ask the owners to donate the fee they would have paid to have their dog euthanised.

All in all, this offer was generally well received, and threw many a dog a much-needed lifeline.

One such dog was Gracie, a stunning two-year-old golden retriever, brought in by one of her owners for euthanasia. Gracie's owners had recently divorced and neither party could come to an agreement on who Gracie should live with. They felt that Gracie was suffering because of their relationship breakdown, and genuinely believed that this was the kindest thing to do. Jenny persuaded Gracie's owners to sign her over. Gracie was successfully rehomed a short time later, to a family that had recently lost their elderly retriever.

Kojak, another dog who was given a second chance, was a personal favourite of mine. A big, clumsy, lout of a dog, Kojak was a mix of all sorts; his black and tan coat suggested some Rottweiler, while his upstanding ears, which tended to flop over every time he tipped his head, hinted at something like a German shepherd. Kojak had a long, fringed tail, capable of bruising your shins if you got caught by it – a common occurrence as it never stopped wagging. At only a year old, and with feet the size of small dinner plates, I wouldn't have been surprised if somewhere along the line, Kojak also had a bit of Great Dane in his ancestry.

Kojak had no manners at all; he loved people, but tended to knock the wind out of them by planting his enormous feet on their chests in an attempt to cover their faces in slobbery licks. He barged about everywhere, always in a rush. Kojak had no regard for who or what stood in his way and often left a trail of devastation wherever he went.

Kojak's owners confessed that they had no idea that the tiny eight-week-old puppy they had acquired from an advert in a local newspaper would grow to such a size. They had a young family and were struggling to cope with his boisterous nature. They admitted that they just didn't have the time or resources to give Kojak what he needed. With no local rescue centres having space for him, Kojak's owners had decided to have him euthanised.

This decision may come as a surprise to you, much as in the case of Gracie. Here were two perfectly healthy dogs facing certain death for no other reason than an owner's belief that there were simply no other options.

Owning a dog is a twelve-year-plus commitment to nuture them from puppy to adulthood and beyond. That commitment also includes making the right decisions for the dog even if that means putting their needs ahead of your own. Building a solid relationship based on trust, understanding, and continued learning is key to maintaining a successful relationship with any dog.

confessions of a veterinary nurse

Gracie nearly lost her life because her owners chose to think what was best for themselves, not what was best for Gracie. Kojak almost lost his because his owners hadn't invested adequate time and effort in him as a puppy. Neither one deserved to die, they were just very badly let down by the people who claimed to love them. Sadly, Gracie and Kojak's stories are not unusual. Every year, countless dogs are euthanised across the UK because they were let down by their owners. Dogs are a privilege to own: they give back tenfold what we give to them. Their love and devotion is unequivocal, and they have the power to brighten the darkest of days. If you've been lucky enough to share your life with a dog, you will understand this completely.

But what happened to Kojak?

After a quiet word with Jenny, a donation was made and Kojak was handed over.

I have to say, I developed a huge soft spot for the clumsy oaf. Kojak's problem was that he really wasn't aware that he was such a big dog. At just under a year old, he was still very much puppy-like in his behaviour, jumping up, mouthing, chewing, and generally getting up to all sorts of mischief. I got used to standing in the back kitchen, looking out of the window, and seeing Jenny go flying past, clinging to Kojak's lead as she desperately tied to teach him some lead skills. We all got used to sporting muddy paw prints on our uniforms, and having to wipe the slobber from our faces and hair. Kojak's clownish antics constantly kept us on our toes.

Jenny spent time with Kojak every day, and started with the basics. She taught him to sit and stay, encouraged him to walk calmly on the lead, and taught him to greet people without the use of his paws. Kojak was a real foodie and responded well to treats as a reward for his good behaviour.

I even took to walking Kojak into town during my lunch breaks. I use the word 'walk' very loosely – I alternated between jogging to keep up with his long, striding steps, and being dragged towards a particularly interesting lamppost or rubbish bin. Kojak loved market day, and quickly became friends with the owner of a pet food stall. Kojak would pull like crazy to get to him, and was always rewarded with a tasty snack or two. One of Kojak's favourite treats was, appropriately enough, a lollipop-shaped hide chew (a homage to his lolly-loving namesake). I would sit on a bench in town, eating my sandwiches, whilst Kojak lay at my feet crunching away on his lolly.

Kojak stayed with us at Greenfields for several weeks, whilst Jenny worked hard on his training and tried to find him a suitable home where it could be continued.

I am a firm believer that there is a dog out there to suit everyone, and in Kojak's case, his perfect match came in the form of a retired police dog handler and his wife.

Kojak, dare I say, looked almost dainty when stood next to this giant bear of a man, whose gruff exterior was in complete contrast to the gentle, caring soul who stepped up and gave our special boy a chance.

I felt a mixture of emotions as Kojak left Greenfields to start his new life, striding effortlessly alongside his new owner, tail held high and swishing as he went. I knew Kojak would be okay, that he had found his forever home. My leaving gift to Kojak was a bag of his favourite lollipop chews.

We received regular updates from Kojak's new family: he settled into his new life straight away, enjoying long country walks, and developing a fondness for pubs and their cuisine, often being allowed to indulge in homemade pies, and even the odd steak or two. And he still got his daily lollipop.

That leaves the question: what about those dogs who somehow fall between the cracks? The ones presented for euthanasia in a poor physical state, who could be restored to full health with nothing more than time and a little tender loving care?

This was exactly the case with Merlin the Dalmatian.

I first met Merlin during one of my afternoon shifts. I had started my shift as usual, with a ward round with the duty vet, Matthew, and Freddie. Together, we ran through the patient list, who had what procedures done, their post-operative instructions and discharge times, etc. In one of the larger kennels, I spotted a very dejected-looking Dalmatian sitting on a blanket, his head drooping so low his chin was almost touching the ground. My heart instantly went out to this poor dog who was in such a sorry state. I had not seen a dog so emaciated in all my life (and to this day still never have). He was little more than a living skeleton.

As I approached his kennel, he lifted his head to look at me, and I heard a thud as his tail thumped on the bottom of his kennel. His eyes, deeply sunk in their sockets, were dull and listless, but his dry, cracked nose did start to twitch a little as I popped my hand through the bars to gently rub the side of his face.

"This is Merlin," said Matthew. "Would you believe he's only eighteen months old?"

I took a deep breath and shook my head in disbelief at this dog who was looking back at me with total defeat etched on his pinched face.

Matthew continued: "it seems that Merlin was bought for an elderly gentleman by members of his family, to keep him company after his wife died, but sadly no-one kept a close eye on either of them. Merlin's owner started having some problems with his memory and simply forgot to feed him. He's now had a bad fall and is being looked after in a care home. None of his family were interested in taking in Merlin, so he was brought here to be euthanised. It's a bit of a kicker, isn't it? The poor dog was literally starving to death. Luckily for us, Jenny managed to get them to sign him over, and I'm sure we can get him right again." Matthew flashed me a quick smile. "Merlin is due for something to eat now; would you like to feed him?"

I didn't need to be asked twice. Knowing how hungry he must be, it was tempting to feed him huge bowls of food, but Matthew advised that Merlin's digestive system simply wouldn't be able to handle it, and that the little-and-often approach was the best way forward.

I opened a tin of dog food and measured a tablespoon into a clean bowl. Merlin could obviously smell the food, and he looked up at me, licking his lips in anticipation.

Carefully opening his kennel door, I sat beside Merlin and placed the bowl in front of him. Whoosh! In a fraction of a second, the food was gone, the bowl licked until it was squeaky clean.

The next thing on the agenda for Merlin was a much-needed bath. It was clear to see from his urine-stained feet and dirt-encrusted coat that Merlin had

Confessions of a veterinary nurse

not had a great deal of outside access. I gathered everything I might need. As we had no animal bathing facilities at Greenfields, I was used to making do with what we had.

I filled a bucket with warm water, grabbed a few clean towels, some cloths, and a bottle of moisturising shampoo. Luckily, it was a warm day, so after leading Merlin outside to my makeshift bathing station, I set to work.

Merlin didn't object at all as I dipped a cloth in the warm water and used it to wet his coat. Now I was in closer contact with Merlin, the smell of stale urine that emanated from him stung my eyes, so much so it made them water, and I had to keep stopping to wipe them. The water that ran off Merlin's coat as I continued to soak him was a dark brown, showing just how much filth was ground into his coat. Once satisfied that Merlin was completely soaked, I applied a small amount of shampoo along his back and began to work it in gently with my fingers. As I started to massage the shampoo in, I became aware of pressure sores on both of his elbows, hocks, and on the top of his hip bones. These were most likely caused by a combination of having too little soft tissue to provide a protective cushion over these joints, and, I suspected, from lying on a hard floor for long periods of time. I was especially careful when cleaning these areas.

Merlin seemed to be enjoying what was probably the first pampering session he'd ever had in his short life. He stood patiently and let out contented little groans when I massaged the shampoo into his shoulders and along his back.

As his muscles were quite weak due to being so malnourished, Merlin was unable to stand for too long, and he lay down at one point on an old blanket I spread out on the ground for him. This enabled me to give his urine-stained feet a really good soak, as well as clip his nails, which were so overgrown one or two had curled around on themselves, which must have been causing Merlin a lot of pain whenever he tried to walk.

Gradually, the snow white of Merlin's coat started to show through the grime, together with his characteristic black spots. Underneath the dirt and grime, he was a handsome boy just waiting to be unleashed.

Once I had rinsed off all the shampoo, I dried Merlin with a clean towel.

During the bathing process, I spoke to Merlin constantly in a reassuring manner. I chattered away to him about how his life was going to change for the better, and that we would find him a new home with someone who would always care for him.

Once dry, I led Merlin back into his kennel, settled him down on top of a thick blanket, and applied a soothing cream to his pressure sores. Merlin accepted all of this with a quiet grace, looking at me quizzically from time to time as if trying to make sense of the sudden change in his circumstances. Having polished off another small meal, Merlin curled up on his blanket, tucked his head under his tail, and dropped into a peaceful sleep. I gave him one last cuddle before leaving him for the night.

And so began Merlin's recovery. Day by day, Merlin grew in strength, as his little-and-often feeding regime began to work its magic.

Vets, nurses, and receptionists alike couldn't help but fall for Merlin's charms – he had such a sweet disposition despite his poor start in life.

There was no 'quick fix' for Merlin, no life-saving drug or complex surgery was required to put this young dog back on his feet again. What Merlin needed was regular feeding, a warm bed, friends who believed in him, and time; and for Merlin, we had all the time in the world.

It was wonderful to watch Merlin's recovery over the following weeks. From a skinny, smelly wretch who had just about given up all hope, Merlin blossomed into a strikingly handsome dog who lit up a room upon entering it. His eyes, once dull and lifeless, sparkled with vitality and energy. Firm muscles rippled under his immaculate coat, which gleamed from his daily brushing sessions, and he single-handedly melted all our hearts with his tongue-lolling smile and non-stop tail wagging.

It was plain to see that Merlin had managed to capture the hearts of all of us at Greenfields, but none more so than Brenda, one of the evening receptionists. Brenda would come in early at the start of each shift to feed Merlin one of his meals, and would also stay behind at the end of her day to settle Merlin for the night.

As far as happy endings go, things couldn't have gone better for Merlin, and after just over six weeks in our care, Merlin left Greenfields to start his new life with Brenda and her family.

There is no better feeling than knowing that you have been instrumental in saving a life and changing it for the better. Jenny taught me so much about how important it is to always try to offer help, a lesson which has never left me. Nowadays, I volunteer for a local dog rescue in my spare time, and I think part of me will never stop looking out for the next Gracie, Kojak, or Merlin.

Visit Hubble and Hattie on the web:
www.hubbleandhattie.com • www.hubbleandhattie.blogspot.co.uk
Details of all books • Special offers • Newsletter • New book news

87

A bird (or cat) in the hand ...

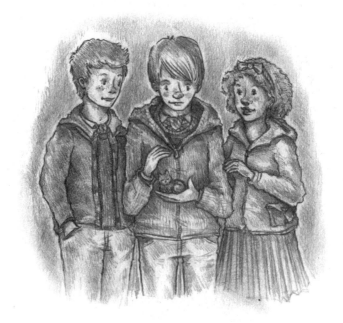

"Okay, so who wants to come out on a visit?"

Always an attention-grabbing statement, it signalled an opportunity to get out and about with the vet, dealing with who knows what. I admit to always being first in line when a shout went out for a willing assistant.

"I need help with an injured swan," muttered Matthew, as he bustled past me into the pharmacy, scanning the shelves before grabbing a bottle of antibiotics and a roll of cotton wool. "Grab your coat and a stitch kit, we're leaving in five minutes."

Did I hear that correctly, I thought, as I watched Matthew striding away – a swan?

Shrugging, I made my way over to the surgical unit, picked up a stitch kit, suture materials, and a container of surgical skin scrub.

Five minutes later, the car was loaded up and we were off.

As he drove, Matthew explained that a call had come through reporting a swan that had been found injured, possibly by a fox, and had lost a lot of blood. The swan was one of a bonded pair that resided at a local country property.

Leaving town behind us, we drove out into the countryside. After following Matthew's map and the directions that we had been given, we eventually turned off the road, made our way up a sweeping gravel driveway, and parked in front of an imposing Georgian-style mansion, in front of which stood a tweed-clad lady waving a handkerchief at us.

Gathering our equipment, we climbed out of the car.

"You must be from the vets?" she asked, clutching the handkerchief and twisting it anxiously in her hands. "It's Swanhilda. She is dreadfully hurt, and I just didn't know what to do. Harold is beside himself."

Matthew laid a reassuring hand on the lady's shoulder. "It's okay," he soothed. "I'm sure we can help. I take it you're Mrs Allard-Smythe?"

"Yes, yes," she replied. "Follow me down to the lake – they're both down there."

To access the lake, which was at the back of the property, we had to skirt around some beautifully manicured lawns, lined with rows of perfectly trimmed topiary shrubs and trees.

Once we were lakeside, we found our patient, sitting quietly, surrounded by bloodied feathers, and looking very sorry for herself. Next to her, another swan (presumably Swanhilda's partner, Harold) was standing protectively over her. As soon as he saw us, Harold drew himself up to his full height and started making low hissing noises.

"Now, now, Harold," said Mrs Allard-Smythe in a quiet but firm voice. "The vet has come to help." She took a few paces forward and began stroking Harold's neck, whispering gently to him. It seemed to have the desired effect, so Matthew and I turned our attention to Swanhilda.

It was plain to see that she was badly injured, and on closer inspection we found several deep wounds on her chest and along the length of her back. Swanhilda was very subdued, and barely moved as we carried out our examination. That in itself was a worry, and suggested that she was also suffering from a degree of shock.

"These wounds are too severe to be stitched here," said Matthew, turning to Mrs Allard-Smythe. "We will have to transport Swanhilda back to the surgery where we can take a proper look at them."

"Do whatever it takes," replied Mrs Allard-Smythe as she continued to pacify Harold. "I can't lose her."

Decision made, Matthew scooped Swanhilda up into his arms (which was no mean feat, swans are large birds), and we made our way back to the car.

I sat in the passenger seat and Matthew deposited Swanhilda onto my lap.

"Now, keep a good hold of her wings, keep them folded against her body. I don't think she will try to move, but just in case," he advised.

Swanhilda felt very cold, so, as we drove back to the practice, Matthew turned on the car's heating to try to warm her up. It seemed to be doing the trick as she began to rock from side to side in my arms.

I didn't so much mind the rocking, I found it to be quite relaxing. However, Swanhilda had decided that she was, in fact, starting to feel quite a bit better, and that it was time to stretch her wings.

With renewed vigour, Swanhilda attempted to stand up and flap her wings.

"Eeeeeekkkkk," I squealed, as my view suddenly became obscured by feathers.

As much as I wanted to, I couldn't hold on to Swanhilda, and she began to give herself a good old shake.

"Hold on!" shouted Matthew, as he pulled into a lay-by.

Too late, I thought. As I said, swans are not small birds, and alarmingly, Swanhilda appeared to be filling the entire front half of the car. Both of her wings had now escaped from my grasp, and Swanhilda apparently wanted to examine them both, stretching them one by one whilst emitting a powerful snorting noise. Swans, when viewed from a distance, always look immaculate, perfectly dressed in snowy white feathers, but the reality is that they carry a lot of mud and less pleasant adornments, which Swanhilda decided to shower me with.

Like warm rain, I could feel splatters of unmentionable material landing on my face and hair, and a particularly pungent odour was also starting to tickle my nostrils. Desperately, I battled on, trying to renew my grip on Swanhilda's wings. Matthew had also thrown himself into the fray, now that he had parked safely, and with the help of an old calving gown he grabbed off the back seat, we managed to re-establish control of our feathered patient by wrapping her up in it.

"Not far to go now," said Matthew, as we drove off again and pulled up at a set of traffic lights.

I didn't dare reply. I just sat completely still, Swanhilda sitting bolt upright facing forwards on my lap, having taken interest in the car in front of us.

Out of the corner of my eye, I spotted a white car pull up alongside us at the traffic lights, sporting all-too-familiar red stripes and the word 'police.'

"Just act normally," I muttered to myself. "Maybe they won't look." I wasn't a hundred per cent sure, but I thought that riding shotgun with a swan on my lap probably wasn't legal.

I couldn't help myself though, and, painfully slowly, trying to keep the rest of my body motionless for fear of disturbing Swanhilda (who now seemed to be completely relaxed), I turned my head towards the police car. At the same moment, Swanhilda also decided to take a closer look, and simultaneously we turned to look at our neighbours.

I registered the look of astonishment on the police officer's face as he stared back at us. I could only imagine that he was mentally searching for rules regarding the safe transport of large birds, and wondering what he should do next.

I, on the other hand, was praying for the lights to change, and after offering the police officer a weak smile, I turned away and tried to sink further down into my seat. Swanhilda continued to fix her new-found friend with a haughty look of disdain.

Mercifully, the lights changed to green and we moved away. I noticed the police car had not, and assumed that the officer was probably still trying to make sense of what he had just seen.

Once back at the practice, we carefully unloaded Swanhilda and took her straight to the surgical unit. A few hours later, with all her wounds cleaned and sutured, Swanhilda was ready to go home and reunite with her partner Harold. She made her return journey safely secured in the back of a horse trailer alongside two of Mrs Allard-Smythe's grooms.

We received a lovely phone call from Mrs Allard-Smythe a few months later to announce a new arrival – a cygnet called Horatio, who she felt had completed her swan family. All three were reported to be thriving.

I do still wonder if that poor policeman ever filed a report on what he witnessed that day – one very bedraggled passenger and a blood-soaked swan – but maybe he thought best not to.

Whenever we ventured out of the practice, we could expect to travel for miles to reach our patients, but on one occasion the patient was literally right on our doorstep.

Greenfields was situated on a main road, close to two large schools. Twice a day during term-time, students would file past the practice in droves. I could imagine many of the students slowing their pace a little, much as I once did, as they walked past the practice, checking the front car park in case anything exciting was happening. Early spring was always the best time to catch a glimpse of the vets at work. The start of spring heralded lambing season, and as well as the large animal vets being dispatched to local farms to help with difficult births, it was also commonplace for farmers to bring their pregnant ewes directly to the practice. The majority of assisted lambings were relatively straightforward; I doubt there is any sweeter sight than that of a newborn lamb taking it first few faltering steps, and many students had been treated to this truly wonderful spectacle. We got to know some of the students who always stopped to say hello if they spotted us. They always expressed a very genuine interest in whatever it was we were doing.

I was surprised, however, to see a small group of them standing at reception early one morning. We were used to them sitting outside now and then, but to see them in the building was a little unexpected.

"Can I help?" I asked.

One of the students was Toby, a frequent visitor. "We've just found this," he said. "He was in the gutter just outside your practice." Toby lifted a cupped hand, in which sat the smallest scrap of a creature. It took a second or two for me to figure out exactly what it was that Toby was holding.

"Goodness me," I exclaimed. "It's a kitten." Soaking wet (for it had been raining overnight) and freezing cold, it was very young, barely more than a few days old.

"We thought it was a baby squirrel at first due to its colour," explained Toby. "We couldn't believe it was a kitten. Can you save it, do you think?"

Gingerly, I lifted the tiny kitten out of Toby's hand. It was motionless and ice-cold. Its blue-grey coat was spattered with muddy rainwater, and I could well believe that Toby and his friends had mistaken it for a rodent. The last thing you would have expected to find at a busy roadside was a newborn kitten, and I wondered how on earth it had ended up there.

"We will certainly try," I replied. "The first thing we need to do is try to warm him up. A kitten of this age shouldn't be away from their mum, as very young kittens can't regulate their own body temperature. I have to be completely honest with you, he (I had managed a quick peek under the kitten's tail to confirm his sex) is a very poorly boy, but we will give him our best shot. If he has survived so far then he must be a fighter."

"Thank you," said Toby. "You guys are just awesome."

"If any of you want to pop in after school to check on him, feel free to do so." The whole group nodded their heads. "And thank you all so much for taking the time to stop and help."

With that, I hurried off to the surgical unit, holding the kitten tightly against me. As I burst into the kennel room, I almost ran into Elaine, who had just finished setting up prep and theatre for the day's operating list.

"Switch the incubator on, would you Elaine? We have a little one who needs help."

Elaine didn't need to be asked twice, and rushed to set up the incubator. I grabbed the nearest towel and wrapped the kitten in it, patting him gently to dry him off.

"I think we need a little kick-start," I murmured to myself. Moving into the prep room, I used my free hand to rummage in one of the drawers until I found a hairdryer. Setting it to a low heat, I moved it back and forth over the kitten. Elaine joined me.

"The incubator is warming up, should be ready in a few minutes, and I've added some bedding. Gosh, is that a kitten? He's tiny," she exclaimed.

I quickly explained where the kitten had come from, and Elaine confessed to being as puzzled as I was about how he had got there.

"Maybe mum was moving the kittens for some reason and this one was dropped along the way," suggested Elaine, using the tip of her index finger to rub the top of the kitten's head.

"Once we get him dry, we need to think about feeding him," I continued.

"Can I do that?" asked Elaine. "I haven't bottle fed a kitten so young before. I would love to try." She took off to find some feeding equipment.

By this time, we were also joined by James, who gave the kitten a quick once-over. Finding no obvious injuries or congenital birth defects (such as a cleft palate, which could have potentially caused the kitten's mother to abandon him), James concluded that the only thing he could prescribe was food, warmth, and a lot of tender loving care. He also confirmed that the kitten was only a few days old. James warned me that, as we didn't know how long the kitten had been lying in the roadside, his chances were pretty slim, but, as ever, we were prepared to give him a chance.

As I continued to pass the hairdryer over the kitten, he started to respond: a little twitch of a front paw, followed by the tiniest of squeaks. I watched as his little rosebud mouth began to open and close – he was hungry!

Elaine returned in due course, armed with everything she needed to feed the kitten. I handed him over, wrapped in a fresh towel. Tucking him under her arm, Elaine offered the kitten the teat of the tiny feeding bottle, which she had filled with a powdered feline replacement milk, carefully made to the correct consistency and temperature.

We could scarcely believe our eyes when the kitten latched on straight away and noisily sucked on it. Elaine broke into a huge smile as she watched the kitten guzzling away. It was more than we could have hoped for, as the kitten drank nearly a full bottle.

Once finished, Elaine dried his face with a corner of the towel before moving on to the next task. Newborn kittens are unable to control their own bladder and bowels and are usually stimulated to toilet by their mum, who would lick them around their lower abdominal area. To mimic this, Elaine rubbed a cotton wool swab soaked in warm water in a circular motion around the kitten's rear end and lower tummy area, and was quickly rewarded with a little squirt of urine.

Feeling a lot more positive about the kitten's future, we placed him in the incubator and covered him with a soft blanket.

"Right then," I turned to face Elaine. "We need to draw up some sort of a feeding rota. He'll need a bottle feed every two hours or so for at least the next ten days. If he survives beyond that, we can start to decrease the number of feeds until he is weaned."

"You won't need a rota," replied Elaine, looking down at the sleeping bundle nestled safely inside the incubator. "I will look after him."

"Are you sure, Elaine? It's going to be hard work and will involve sleepless nights and potentially a lot of heartbreak if he doesn't make it."

"I am positive," said Elaine, with determination in her voice. "I have a good feeling about this kitten. He is going to be just fine."

True to her word, Elaine devoted herself to caring for the little orphaned kitten. She named him Smokey, due to his very distinctive blue-grey coat. Every morning she would turn up for her shift with her little charge secured in his special padded cat carrier, and would pop him into the incubator where she could keep a close eye on him. Elaine fed him at the times she'd scheduled on the feeding chart she'd made, and she kept him scrupulously clean. Each day that passed, Smokey grew stronger and stronger, and we marked each milestone with undisguised joy: the first time Smokey managed to take his first proper steps on his sturdy little legs, the day his eyes began to open, and the day he started to lap some milk formula from a bowl.

As well as capturing the hearts of everyone in the practice, Smokey had also acquired a fan club, with Toby and friends often calling in to check on his progress.

Most heart-warming of all was the bond that quickly grew between Elaine and Smokey. Smokey loved to sleep snuggled in her arms, and we got used to the tiny cries coming from the incubator whenever he heard Elaine's voice, because he knew he would soon be scooped up and cuddled. It was a bond that endured for fifteen long, happy years, based on total love and devotion from both sides. Smokey touched all our hearts, and will always be fondly remembered as the kitten who defied the odds and survived.

Visit Hubble and Hattie on the web:
www.hubbleandhattie.com • www.hubbleandhattie.blogspot.co.uk
Details of all books • Special offers • Newsletter • New book news

Saving Brock

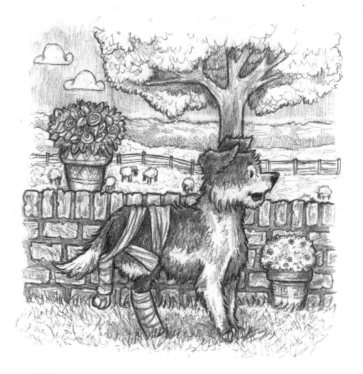

I would not like to hazard a guess at just how many patients I have nursed back to health over the years. From the neonates – vulnerable puppies and kittens, some only hours old – needing a helping hand to get started in life, to those needing a gentle, guiding hand during the final part of their journey, and all the characters in between.

Nursing a patient during my training years was very much a hands-on process. We didn't have modern technology, with all its whistles and bells, to provide us with detailed information about how our patient was faring: we made do with our eyes and ears, and utilised our practical skills to the best of our ability. Some cases tested every one of these skills, and acted as a reminder that where there is life there is always hope. These were the patients who needed us the most.

If you speak to any veterinary professional, they will likely tell you there is one patient whose plight touched their heart in such a way that they are impossible to forget. For me, that patient was a dog called Brock.

Brock was a black and white working Border Collie who belonged to John Sullivan, a local farmer. Brock led an idyllic life on the farm, spending his days either out in the fields running alongside the tractors as they toiled, or rounding up the dozens of sheep scattered across many acres of land. I had been out to the farm where Brock lived several times, to assist the vets, and was always made to feel very welcome. As soon as we got out of the car, Brock would come hurtling over and roll straight onto his back, all four legs pedalling furiously in the air until he got a tummy rub. Brock also had his own signature smile, curling back his lips to expose his pearly white teeth whilst emitting a deep rumbling growl. I could imagine that any stranger visiting the farm may have been a little perturbed by the sight of Brock in full flight, heading their way with his teeth bared, but we knew Brock for what he was: a big soft lump with a heart of gold.

I remember clearly the day it happened: I was sitting on reception, catching up with a bit of paperwork, when suddenly the front door burst open and I heard a loud cry for help.

Two of the farm hands from Sullivan's Farm came crashing through the door. Between them, they were carrying an old fence panel (obviously fashioned into a makeshift stretcher), and lying on top of it, completely motionless, was Brock.

I jumped out of my chair and ushered them into the nearest consulting room.

"I need some help in here!" I shouted at the top of my voice in the hope that someone was nearby. The clattering sound of someone rushing down the stairs moments later confirmed that help was indeed on its way.

The farmhands put the stretcher on the consulting room table and stood back. Both looked shocked and deeply upset.

"Tell me what happened," I said.

"Brock was in one of the barns," said one of the men, who introduced himself as Bill. "He was probably hunting for rats – he's a great rat catcher, is our Brock. He must have gone behind the stack of heavy metal containers that's in the corner, and they toppled over. Brock was trapped underneath. We heard him crying out at first and had to lift the containers off him, but he hasn't made a sound since we moved him."

My mind was whirring with a potential list of injuries that Brock could have sustained, from bone fractures and organ damage to life-threatening internal bleeding.

Whilst waiting for help, I conducted a quick first aid survey, following the ABC protocol for emergency cases: airway, breathing and circulation. Lifting Brock's top lip, I noted that his gums were deathly pale, which indicated that Brock was in a state of shock. It could also mean that he was bleeding internally. Brock's breathing was rapid and shallow, and the extremities of his limbs were cool to the touch – another indicator of shock, as Brock's circulation was currently focussed on more critical parts of his body. I grabbed a stethoscope and listened to his heart. Brock's heart rate was rapid and strangely muffled. I made a mental note of this. There were no obvious external injuries, but from the angle of one of Brock's hind legs, I suspected a fracture.

I called Brock's name softly to assess his level of response and was rewarded with a feeble wag of his tail. Brock was still with us, but it was clear that he was in a very bad way.

After what seemed like an eternity (but was probably only a minute or two), Matthew arrived. I quickly ran through what had happened to Brock and listed my primary observations.

confessions of a veterinary nurse

I knew that time was of the essence, so I excused myself and ran over to the surgical unit to prepare the intravenous fluids I knew Brock would need as the first stage of his treatment. The fluid would hopefully combat the circulatory shock that Brock was suffering from. In a matter of minutes, I had assembled a bag of intravenous fluids and attached to it a fluid administration line. I had gathered an intravenous catheter, a cotton wool swab soaked in surgical spirit (to clean the site on Brock's foreleg where the catheter would go), and a selection of dressing materials to secure the catheter in place. I checked that the surgical clippers were clean and switched on at the mains.

"Right," I said out loud. "We are ready to go."

As soon as I had uttered the words, I heard the door to the surgical unit open and Matthew came in with the two farm hands behind him, Brock still on his makeshift stretcher. Carefully, they rested it on the prep room table.

"Thank you," said Matthew. "You can leave Brock with us now. I will give Mr Sullivan a call a little later when we know more. Tell him we'll do our best for Brock."

Once the farm hands had left, Matthew quickly outlined his plan. He had already administered a heavy dose of pain relief to ensure that Brock was kept as comfortable as possible. Matthew's main concerns were Brock's breathing and his muffled heartbeat, so he wanted to X-ray Brock's chest as a priority. As he was explaining, Matthew clipped a small area of fur away from one of Brock's forelegs, swabbed it several times, and swiftly inserted an intravenous catheter. Once safely secured by surgical tapes, Matthew connected the catheter to the fluid administration line and started the fluids running. It was always reassuring to see the steady drip of the life-saving liquid as it made its way down the plastic tubing and into the patient.

The next step the X-ray. As Brock was so quiet and seemingly unable to move, we managed this without the need for sedation or anaesthesia, which would have been far too risky at this stage. Emergency survey X-rays were often not the best quality but were usually adequate for initial diagnostics.

We took a series of what we liked to call 'dog-o-grams,' trying to capture as many parts of the dog's body as possible. Not having the benefit of today's digital X-rays, which are ready to be viewed within minutes, our X-rays had to be developed manually. In a dedicated dark room, the X-ray films were removed from special cassettes, clipped into metal hangers, then dipped into large containers of developing fluids for set periods of time. Once dipped, the images would develop on the films, and would be rinsed and dried before viewing. All in all, a time-consuming process, and for emergency cases, it was prudent to try to fit as much of the patient onto each film as possible.

It may not have been terribly scientific, but it invariably got us the initial answers that we needed.

In Brock's case, we managed to get some reasonable views of his front and hind legs, his abdomen and his chest.

Our first suspicions were confirmed – Brock had sustained a fracture to his left hind tibia, or shin bone as it's commonly known. It was a clean break that would lend itself to surgical repair. However, the X-rays revealed that Brock had also dislocated his right hip, which required immediate attention to put right. If not relocated quickly, the structures that supported the hip joint and kept the ball of the joint in the socket could become permanently damaged.

The next image clipped onto the illuminated X-ray viewer box on the wall of the prep room was of Brock's chest. As he looked at it, Matthew drew a sharp intake of breath. Chest X-rays usually clearly show the rib cage, lungs and heart, but in Brock's case the heart and lungs were completely obscured. But by what? I had no idea, and had to ask Matthew to elaborate.

"Brock has a diaphragmatic hernia," Matthew explained. "The crushing injury has resulted in a tear in his diaphragm. The diaphragm, as well as playing a part in normal respiration, separates the abdominal contents from the chest cavity. The tear in Brock's diaphragm has allowed some of his abdominal contents to enter his chest. This means that Brock's lungs cannot expand fully, hence his breathing difficulties and his muffled heartbeat." Matthew ran his hand through his hair. "For Brock to have any sort of a chance we need to move back the abdominal organs that have passed into Brock's chest and fix the tear. It's going to be a risky procedure, and I'll need a good assistant anaesthetist on hand." Matthew tipped me a cheeky wink. "First things first, though, we need to stabilise Brock's fractured leg and try to get his dislocated hip back in place."

I had been monitoring Brock closely whilst his X-rays were taken. His gum colour was beginning to improve, his limbs were warming up, and he was becoming a little more responsive, lifting his head now and then to look at his new surroundings. The intravenous fluids were obviously reversing the circulatory shock which was excellent news.

After placing Brock in a kennel that I'd pre-prepared with extra layers of comfortable bedding, Matthew sat down to discuss a treatment and nursing care plan for Brock. We were joined at this point by Jenny, Freddie and Elaine. Between us we would be caring for Brock over the following days.

Clearly, Brock's most serious injury was the damage to his diaphragm, but that did not necessarily mean that it was going to take priority. Brock would need to be stable clinically before surgery was attempted, to minimise some of the risk involved. The dislocated hip did need to be attended to fairly quickly, to give it the best chance of staying put once replaced. The fractured leg, although serious, could at least be stabilised temporarily by the application of a sturdy support bandage, until such time that it could be surgically repaired.

From a nursing point of view, Brock would need to be kept as comfortable as possible: he would need to receive daily pain relief administered by injection, he would need to be turned regularly on his bedding to prevent any pressure sores from forming, his bedding would need to be checked and changed frequently to prevent it from becoming soiled. Initially, Brock was likely to be pretty much immobile, and would need assistance getting up and moving. Brock's food and water intake would also have to be closely monitored to ensure that he was getting adequate fluid and nutrition.

Matthew told me he would review Brock in a few hours. If his vital signs continued to improve, he would consider administering a short anaesthetic to replace Brock's dislocated hip, and would also apply a support dressing to his fractured leg. Matthew left to give Brock's owners a call to discuss the findings and the proposed treatment plan.

That gave me a little time to spend with Brock. Sitting next to him as he lay in his kennel, I spoke softly to him whilst scratching him behind the ears (something I knew Brock loved). I was encouraged to see Brock respond. Brock was such an intelligent dog: lifting his head and resting it on my lap, looking up at me with his trusting eyes, he knew we were there to help him.

Later that afternoon, Matthew checked on Brock's progress. Brock was now quite alert, responding to his name when called, his temperature was within normal range, and he had even started wagging his tail with a bit more enthusiasm. Matthew was confident that Brock could cope with a short anaesthetic, and I held Brock securely in my arms as he drifted off to sleep.

Replacing a dislocated hip isn't the most elegant of procedures, there is a lot of physical force involved to get the ball of the hip back into its socket and there was a bit of a tug of war before we heard the distinct click of the hip popping back into place. Once the hip was back where it should have been, the trick was to keep it there whilst the surrounding support structures healed. At the time, the best method of achieving this was to apply an Ehmer sling to the affected limb.

An Ehmer sling is a notoriously difficult bandage to apply, as it requires the affected leg to be flexed at the knee with the paw rotated slightly inwards, which would then cause the dog's hock joint to rotate outwards. The net effect was that it would hold the ball of the hip firmly in place whilst it healed. The classic figure of eight bandage required a great deal of accuracy and precision. For a trainee nurse, it represented the perfect opportunity to test my bandaging skills.

After setting out an array of different bandaging materials, I set to work. Matthew supported Brock's leg in the correct position as I began to apply different layers of the bandage: starting with a layer of soft padding material, I began to form my figure of eight, adding additional layers of crepe knit bandage to strengthen the bandage and support the limb, before finishing with a covering of robust, adhesive bandage to ensure the limb did not move from its now fixed position. I stood back to admire my handiwork.

"Good work," said Matthew. "We need to keep this on for at least a week. The nursing team will need to ensure that it stays clean and dry, and that it's checked regularly to make sure it doesn't slip or rub against Brock's skin and make it sore. Next job, I think a Robert Jones bandage will keep Brock's fractured leg stable and comfortable until we can repair it."

Another classic dressing: a Robert Jones bandage. This was a thick, multi-layered dressing (which included the use of a whole roll of cotton wool in most cases), designed to provide maximum comfort and support to injured limbs. The measure of a good Robert Jones bandage was to flick the bandage with your fingers once applied. If your flick gave off the same resonance as when flicking a ripe melon, you were onto a winner (and yes, I had spent time furtively skulking around our local fruit and vegetable shops flicking numerous melons to familiarise myself with the sound, much to the surprise and curiosity of my fellow shoppers). This bandage also required a fair amount of skill to ensure it provided the correct level of support: too loose and it would slip, too tight and it could potentially compromise circulation to the entire limb.

Fifteen minutes later, my job was complete. With a few flicks from myself and Matthew, we concurred that the Robert Jones dressing was perfect. As with the Ehmer sling, this bandage required regular checking to ensure that it remained clean and comfortable.

Between us, we carried Brock back to his padded kennel and I stayed with him as he recovered from his anaesthetic. As with all the patients I have ever nursed, I spoke to him quietly as he started to regain consciousness, reassuring him that all had gone well and that we were doing our best to fix him. Brock knew I was there and as soon as he was able to, he started to lick the back of my hand. His way, I am sure, of saying thank you.

Over the next few days, Brock was looked after by the nursing team. After forty-eight hours, he no longer needed the support of intravenous fluids, as he was able to lap water by himself and was also allowing us to hand feed him. As he was still fairly immobile due to the bandages on his hind legs, we had to work in pairs to help Brock stand and go outside to toilet. We fashioned a sling out of a rolled-up bath towel and passed this under Brock's tummy, holding the ends of the towel together over his back. This enabled us to lift Brock comfortably into a standing position. Then, with one person guiding from the front, the nurse holding the sling walked at Brock's side, supporting the weight of his back end. Even though Brock should have been able to use his left hind leg to walk on, he chose not to and seemed perfectly at ease with being assisted. We were keen to do whatever suited Brock, to ensure he remained as stress-free as possible. This helped keep his breathing relaxed, especially important since his chest was still full of things that really shouldn't have been there, and his lungs were still not able to fully inflate. Whilst he was in a standing position, we took the time to check Brock's dressings, making sure they were still in place and had not become soiled. We also checked him over thoroughly. As Brock was spending most of his time lying down, it was important to ensure that he did not develop any pressure sores. Once we had checked his skin, Brock had a pamper session with a brush and comb to ensure that his dense coat remained in tip-top condition and tangle free. Clinical checks were also carried out daily and recorded on his hospitalisation sheet. The nursing team checked and recorded Brock's temperature, pulse, and respiration rate twice a day. As Brock was a dog used to living life in the fast lane, it was also important to keep him mentally stimulated. I took to bringing my nurse training notes in to read to him during my lunch breaks. Two of us would carry him, using his sling, out to the back garden, and lie him on a blanket so he could enjoy a bit of fresh air and a change of scenery. I would eat my lunch beside him, telling him all about the skeletal, muscular and circulatory systems of the mammalian body. I swear he took in every word I said. I also shared my lunch with him, breaking off bits of my sandwich and playing a game: I would put a bit of sandwich in one hand and close my fist around it, offer both hands to Brock, and he would have to let me know which hand the tit-bit was in by nudging it with his nose. Brock, being a collie, soon got the hang of it.

For patients, mental stimulation is an integral part of any recovery. Adopting a holistic approach to nursing, ie treating the patient as a whole instead of just focusing on a list of injuries or disease symptoms, can have a positive impact on recovery times. Brock was a working dog, with a mind as agile as his body, and it was important that we did not lose sight of that.

Confessions of a veterinary nurse

* * *

Five days later, Matthew decided that Brock was stable enough to undergo the tricky surgery to repair the tear in his diaphragm. We had kept the whole day free so that Brock would have our undivided attention. As this procedure was quite an unusual one, there was no shortage of nurses offering their help. I was the nominated anaesthetic monitoring nurse, Freddie had offered to 'scrub in' as an assistant, to provide a spare pair of hands to pass instruments as they were required, and Elaine was on hand to continually monitor Brock's vital signs throughout the procedure.

Together, we set up the surgical theatre, checking and double checking that everything was in order and close at hand. Before we began, we had a team meeting to discuss our separate roles and how they would work together, and after a strong cup of coffee we were ready to go.

I think we were all feeling a little nervous and apprehensive as we carried an anaesthetised Brock into theatre and prepped him for surgery.

My sole objective during the procedure was literally to breathe for Brock. Once Matthew was in a position to carefully extract Brock's abdominal contents from within his chest cavity, it was crucial that his lungs were able to inflate properly and regularly whilst the tear in his diaphragm was repaired, as Brock would be unable to do this for himself. I sat on a chair next to Brock's head, my brow furrowed in concentration as I timed each squeeze of the breathing bag that formed part of Brock's anaesthetic circuit. Fresh oxygen was delivered by continuous flow via a full oxygen tank that was attached to the back of the anaesthetic machine. Mixed with an anaesthetic agent, this life-giving oxygen was keeping Brock both alive and safely anaesthetised. A snug-fitting breathing tube had been passed into Brock's windpipe once he was asleep, which was then connected to the anaesthetic circuit, to allow an unobstructed flow of gas into Brock's lungs.

Whilst I focused on squeezing the breathing bag, Elaine watched Brock's vital signs, recording them on a monitoring sheet. Even though there were four of us in the compact theatre, the silence was only broken by the steady whooshes of gas as I squeezed the oxygen bag, and the metallic tinkle of surgical instruments as they were placed on the surgical trolley. The only time anyone spoke was in response to one of Elaine's questions about Brock's level of anaesthesia. Nowadays, for procedures such as this, there are mechanical ventilators to accurately deliver calculated volumes of oxygen into the lungs, pulse oximeters to measure oxygen saturation, capnography to measure how much carbon dioxide is present in the patient's breath – an invaluable tool when it comes to assessing respiration – ECG, blood pressure monitors, and a dizzying array of tools to help safely maintain and monitor an anaesthetised patient. We had little more than a simple recording chart, our own eyes and ears, and the training, knowledge, and confidence to do our utmost to keep our patients safe, which was exactly what Brock needed from us.

After what seemed like the longest time, Matthew set down the last of his instruments on the nearby trolley, took off his protective face mask, and peeled off his surgical gloves.

"So far so good," he said. "I have repaired the tear. It should be good and strong. Now it's down to you, Brock."

Once again, I found myself kneeling beside Brock as he slowly woke up. Cradling his head in my arms, I spoke to him, delivering the same calm reassurance that I had done since the start of Brock's journey. I stayed with him until he was fully awake and able to lap a small amount of water from a bowl that I held under his nose. Watching the steady rise and fall of Brock's chest, I felt a rush of relief and elation wash over me. It was pleasing to see that Brock's lungs were inflating well because it meant that the repair to his diaphragm was holding.

I was reluctant to leave Brock that night, finding lots of extra cleaning jobs to do, giving me the perfect opportunity to keep popping my head into his kennel to see how he was faring. However, I finally called it a day when, much to my relief, I spotted Jenny walking across to the surgical unit, dragging a sleeping bag behind her. I knew full well what that meant: Brock was going to have his very own night nurse.

For the next three nights, Jenny slept next to Brock to ensure that he wasn't left unattended. Brock had been through major thoracic surgery, and we were all keen to ensure that his recovery went as smoothly as possible.

I do believe that Brock loved all the attention he was getting. We all fussed around him like mother hens around a chick. Whether it was hand feeding him delicate morsels of tasty food (most of which seemed to come from our own lunch boxes), or plumping up his bedding, or just stopping by to give him an ear scratch, Brock quickly built himself an army of devoted followers, willing to cater to his every whim. We continued to use a body sling to take Brock outside at least twice a day; he was still not interested in walking himself and seemed perfectly at ease being carried about, although theoretically, he should have been able to walk by himself. One of his hind legs was still being held off the ground in the Ehmer sling, but the other, although well encased by a bulky dressing was more than able to support his weight. It seemed that Brock simply didn't want to walk by himself just yet.

I loved spending my lunch breaks with Brock. I laid a padded bed at the bottom of the garden, and with some help, Brock would be settled down on it. After sharing my sandwiches with him, I would sit and chat or read to him from one of my study books. Sometimes, we would just sit and listen to the birds singing and the rustle of the surrounding trees as the wind blew gently through them. I always took a brush with me and groomed Brock's coat until it shone. I would often hand over to either Jenny, Freddie, or Elaine, who would also sit with Brock and share their lunch with him. When it was time to bring Brock in, we tried to encourage him to walk, even just a few steps. After helping him into a standing position, one of us would stand a short distance away and call him. Brock would respond by pricking up his ears and tipping his head quizzically to one side, his tail wagging steadily, but still, he refused to budge, and we resorted to carrying him.

Matthew continued to check him twice a day, and could come up with no reasonable explanation as to why Brock wouldn't take those first few steps, but assured us that he would in his own sweet time.

It was a week after his thoracic surgery, and I was just settling down with Brock in the back garden when I realised I'd forgotten to pick up my sandwiches. There was no one around to watch Brock for me, but as he had shown no interest whatsoever in moving from his bed once he was settled, I felt confident that he'd be okay whilst I quickly got my lunch.

"Be a good boy, Brock. Stay," I said, ruffling the fur around his neck.

I took a quick look behind me as I opened the door to the main building: Brock hadn't moved but was watching me intently.

It took me a couple of minutes to grab my sandwiches, and I rushed back to Brock. I'm certain my heart froze when I spotted the empty bed - Brock was nowhere to be seen! Panic-stricken –and trying to hide it from my voice - I called his name. I almost swooned when, out of the corner of my eye, I saw the tip of Brock's bushy tail under a hedge. And glory be, there he stood! He looked very proud of himself, having clearly got up and walked over to a patch of shade. The sun was quite warm that day, and Brock had obviously decided he needed to cool down. And to top it off, when I called his name and he turned to face me, he was wearing his unique smile! I hadn't seen Brock smile since his accident, but there he was, lips rolled back, exposing his teeth in the widest, goofiest grin I had ever seen.

"And what do you think you are doing, young man?" I asked sternly, hands on my hips. Brock responded by slowly hopping towards me, maintaining his toothy grin.

Once he reached me, Brock dropped, somewhat clumsily, to the ground and rolled onto his back, the hind leg encased inside the heavy Robert Jones dressing sticking straight up in the air like a flagpole.

"Have you been having us on, Brock?" I murmured, squatting down to rub the tummy that had been so graciously offered, I am sure, as a peace offering.

"I think you have been able to walk all along, cheeky boy."

Facing Brock, I stood up, took a few steps backwards and called his name. Brock managed to flip himself upright, using his bandaged leg to push himself up (bearing in mind his other hind leg was folded against his body inside the sling), and once again he hopped over to me, looking very pleased with this newly acquired skill.

"Well," I said. "I don't think we'll use the body sling to get you back inside today. Are you going to follow me then?"

Slowly, I continued walking backwards so I could watch Brock's progress, making my way into the surgical unit, Brock maintaining a steady pace to keep up with me.

Once inside I called out: "come and see Brock, everyone!"

Matthew and Elaine popped their heads around the corner and their faces lit up with delight when they saw Brock walking proudly towards them, completely unaided.

"Way to go, Brock," exclaimed Matthew, stooping to gather Brock in a warm hug. "I knew you could do it."

That was Brock's turning point. From that day, there was no stopping him. When we let him out of his kennel in the mornings, he would hop his way joyfully down the garden, and happily sniff about for a while, enjoying the fresh air. Once we had finished our daily operation list, we let him to potter about in the prep room whilst we cleaned, as he so enjoyed the company and chatter. Matthew decided that the Ehmer sling had been on long enough, and that, since Brock was doing so well, it was time to repair his fractured leg.

With a feeling of déjà vu, I held Brock as he was anaesthetised once more, hopefully for the last time. The surgery to repair Brock's leg was relatively straightforward. A metal plate was fixed onto his tibia by several screws, which effectively held the fractured ends of bone together to allow them to heal. Another Robert Jones dressing was applied to support the limb during the early stages of healing. Matthew removed Brock's Ehmer sling and took some post-operative X-rays to ensure that everything was as it should be. There was a collective sigh of relief from us all as I clipped Brock's X-rays onto the viewer. Not only was the fracture repair looking rock solid with the bones in perfect alignment, but Brock's right hip had also remained in place. Overall, they were the best results we could have hoped for. All Brock needed now was time and rest to allow Mother Nature to work her magic.

It was four months later when Matthew and I drove up the long farm track to Sullivan's Farm. All the time I was scanning the surroundings looking for that one familiar face.

I wasn't disappointed. As we climbed out of the car, I spotted Brock in the distance about the same time he spotted us.

We stood and marvelled as Brock galloped towards us at full speed, all four legs moving with ease, without a trace of lameness. As he got within a few hundred yards of us, Brock broke into his infamous smile, following it up with a long, melodious growl. Literally skidding to a halt at our feet, Brock threw himself down and spun over onto his back, legs pistoning away in the air: how could we resist? We were well and truly putty in his paws.

As he nuzzled into my outstretched hand, I looked into Brock's intelligent eyes, which sparkled with health and vitality, and I knew that this dog understood, without any doubt, that we had saved his life. And by that act, we had created an unbreakable bond; a little piece of my heart will now always belong to Brock – the collie who learned to smile again.

Visit Hubble and Hattie on the web:
www.hubbleandhattie.com • www.hubbleandhattie.blogspot.co.uk
Details of all books • Special offers • Newsletter • New book news

Ending an era

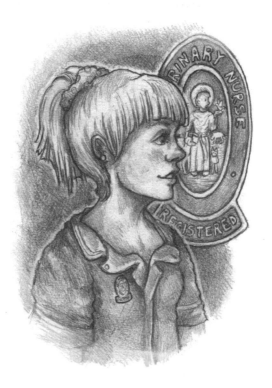

Brock's story pretty much sums up the role of a veterinary nurse. From the second an emergency case crashes through the door, instinct, medical knowledge, empathy, and a wide range of other skills are automatically deployed. Veterinary nurses, much as their human counterparts, are the caregivers, the ones keeping a cool head no matter what challenges are presented to them. An old saying in the veterinary profession is that 'behind every good vet there is an equally good nurse.' It's a symbiotic relationship based on mutual respect and the need to do the very best for the patients in ourr care.

Our job wasn't all about cuddling fluffy kittens and snuggling puppies, as could often be the perception. Our job was a tough one. Every day we were faced with difficult decisions, every day we had to deal with the emotional impact that having a sick or injured pet had on their owners, and every day we strived to help in any way that we could to make things better for all concerned.

Our patients sometimes didn't appreciate all that we were trying to do for them. I have been bitten, scratched, kicked, pecked, squashed, and trampled. I have scars both physical and emotional that will stay with me for the rest of my life. I've had plenty of sleepless nights wondering if I had done enough, or if I could have altered an outcome. I take comfort in knowing that I am not alone, and for the countless veterinary nurses out there that toss and turn each night, always remember that you are part of something truly wondrous, a way of life that few people outside of the profession will ever truly understand. Remember that your dedication, courage, and compassion will always shine through, the brightest of beacons to lighten the darkest of days.

And what of those who support us on our chosen path? The families and friends who lie awake worrying, as we set off into the night to assist with an urgent cas; those who sit at home waiting for us to come home, late again because we needed to stay behind to help; the ones who offer a shoulder to cry on when our day has been full of heartbreak. They are the true heroes, because without them we couldn't do what we do, and for that, I salute them all.

I will always be grateful for the opportunity to be part of the veterinary world. I have made many lifelong friends; friends who truly understand who I am and what drives me. Together, we have shared tears and laughter, and every success and failure, because, after all, we are only human.

It was a proud day indeed when, after passing my second-year exams, I pinned my official badge, issued by The Royal College of Veterinary Surgeons, onto my brand new (and very modern) bottle green uniform. Bearing the title Veterinary Nurse (a recent change from the previous Animal Nursing Auxiliary title) and depicting an image of St Francis of Assisi, patron saint of animals, I felt an overwhelming sense of achievement. Two years of hard study had paid off: another day of cream cakes, and another neatly typed letter from Mr Crossland. This was where I belonged; this was my dream come true. A dream that was to last for thirty years.

I remained at Greenfields for several years, being promoted to Head Nurse following Jenny's departure, when she left to move closer to her elderly mother. Initially, I felt a little out of my depth in my new role. Jenny's years of experience meant that I had big shoes to fill, but I was supported from day one by Freddie and Elaine, and the team of vets and receptionists, something that I will be eternally thankful for. As the years flew by, my confidence continued to grow, and I started to feel worthy of the badge I wore every day. I knew that Jenny would be proud of me, and that's all that mattered.

When I was 21, I decided to stretch my wings, and accepted the position of Head Nurse at a new mixed practice on the other side of town. Feeling like a proper grown-up now – I was engaged to my future husband and we had taken our first step on the property ladder – I relished the prospect of a new challenge. The new practice had opened two years earlier, and was pretty much still in its infancy. I missed my Greenfields colleagues so much initially, I almost regretted my decision to move, but at Meadowside Vets I found a whole new set of lifelong friends.

Over the next few years, I worked closely with my new practice principal, Stuart, a vet, and his wife, Christine, who were a level-headed, no-nonsense couple with a flair for business. Together, we developed Meadowside into a successful and thriving practice. Stuart and Christine were very family-orientated, and treated every member of staff as one of their own. I quickly settled into my role, and worked hard to ensure that the practice blossomed.

confessions of a veterinary nurse

Of course, there were many adventures along the way, highs and lows, ups and downs, but we were a strong team and we always pulled together.

The time seemed to fly by, and before I knew it, I had chalked up thirty years of dedicating my life to improving the welfare of animals.

The veterinary profession is changing at a dizzying pace: advanced technology, scientific breakthroughs, and ground-breaking surgical procedures are a far cry from our rather more haphazard days of 'giving it a go and seeing what happens,' but I look back on those days with an immense feeling of fondness and sense of pride. We lived by our wits, relied on our gut feelings, and, even more so, relied on each other.

Even though I retired from veterinary nursing in 2018, I have found it difficult to let go, spending my days volunteering at a local dog rescue centre, and becoming one of the trustees. I help fundraise with a small group of friends and our dogs. I also visit local care homes with Scout, one of my current rescue dogs, as a volunteer for Pets As Therapy, a UK charitable organisation helping to provide people with the unequivocal love and companionship that dogs are so skilled at delivering.

I can also be found, once a month or so, in a local hostelry enjoying a good old catch up and a pub quiz with Freddie and Elaine, both of whom are still working in the profession. Freddie has more than a little sprinkling of silver in his pesky beard now, and Elaine and I like to spend time comparing the growing number of grey streaks in our own hair. We grumble about our aches and pains and reminisce about times gone by. There is something curiously unspoken and wonderful about the bond between us, an invisible one that can never be broken.

Together we made a difference; together we saved lives.

A life less ordinary? You can be the judge of that.

Another great book from Tracey Ison:

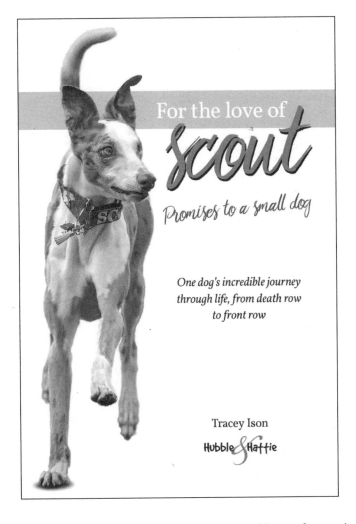

When Tracey and Paul adopted Scout, they promised him safety and security, and a life free from fear and loneliness: all the things denied him during his first few months of life. Discover how Scout's carers learned to build on the unconditional trust and devotion that this clumsy, flat-footed, loveable Lurcher offered.

ISBN: 978-1-845849-36-8
Paperback • 22.5x15.2cm • 112 pages • 47 colour pictures • £8.99

For more information and price details, visit our website at www.hubbleandhattie.com
• email: info@hubbleandhattie.com • Tel: +44(0)1305 260068

Say hello to Hubble & Hattie Kids!

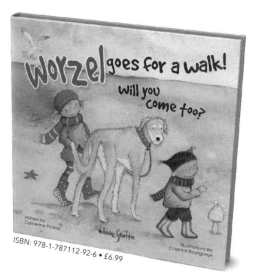

ISBN: 978-1-787112-92-6 • £6.99

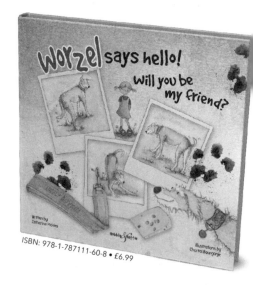

ISBN: 978-1-787111-60-8 • £6.99

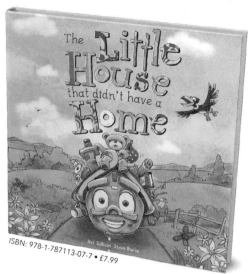

ISBN: 978-1-787113-07-7 • £7.99

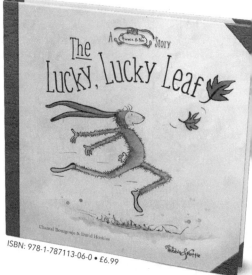

ISBN: 978-1-787113-06-0 • £6.99

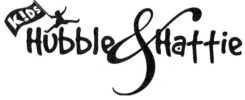

The latest addition ...

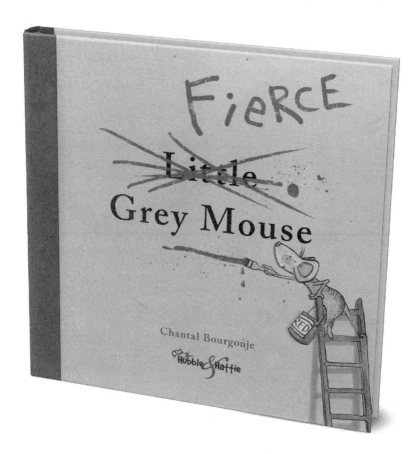

In a world full of happy, fluffy animals, ONE Mouse wants to be FIERCE. He exercises, eats mountains of porridge and drinks lots of milk. He practises his roaring and pouncing skills. Soon, Little Grey Mouse is Fierce Grey Mouse. But what happens when his friends want to play with Little Grey Mouse and find only Fierce Grey Mouse ...?

ISBN: 978-1-787113-12-1
Hardback • 20.5x20.5cm • 32 pages • £6.99

For more information and price details, visit our website at www.hubbleandhattie.com
• email: info@hubbleandhattie.com • Tel: +44(0)1305 260068

New from Hubble & Hattie:

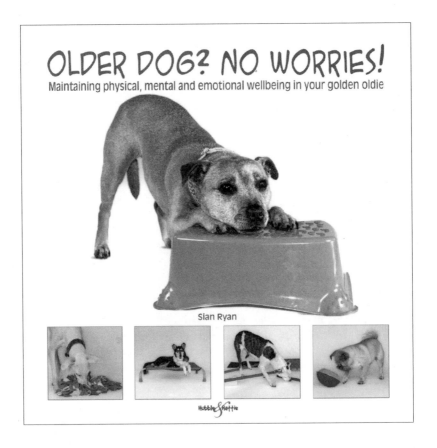

Everything you need to know to maximise quality of life for your older dog.
Offering advice and ideas for mental, physical, and emotional support as your
dog ages and his needs change, including the latest research, and designed
to help you create a bespoke care plan for your dog.

ISBN: 978-1-787113-66-4
Paperback • 20.5x20.5cm • 96 pages • 100 pictures • £13.99

For more information and price details, visit our website at www.hubbleandhattie.com
• email: info@hubbleandhattie.com • Tel: +44(0)1305 260068

Index

Visit Hubble and Hattie on the web:
www.hubbleandhattie.com • www.hubbleandhattie.blogspot.co.uk
Details of all books • Special offers • Newsletter • New book news